WELLBEING THROUGH FOOD & DISCIPLINE

THE CHATURMASA DIARIES

Compiled & Edited
By

AJAY, MAHESH, RAJESH, VP AND VIVEK

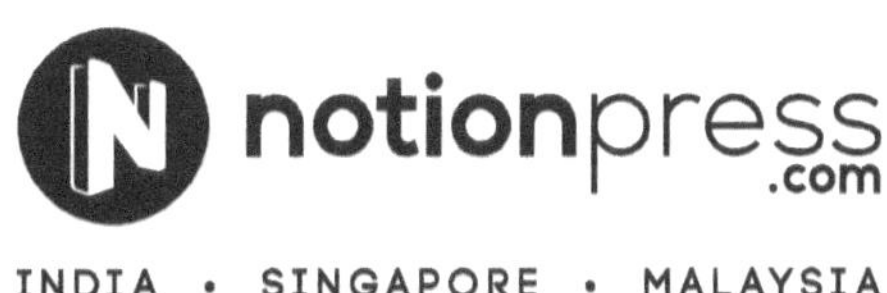

Notion Press Media Pvt Ltd

No. 50, Chettiyar Agaram Main Road,
Vanagaram, Chennai, Tamil Nadu – 600 095

First Published by Notion Press 2021
Copyright © Ajay, Mahesh, Rajesh, VP and Vivek 2021
All Rights Reserved.

ISBN 978-1-63940-351-6

Table of Contents

Acknowledgements & Gratitude

No initiative, especially one as difficult as lifestyle changes and inner transformation ever succeeds without contribution from several people. We are eternally grateful first of all to the entire *guru parampara* and practitioners who have preserved the eternal knowledge and wisdom in the form of scriptures and are ever ready to help a novice get on the path. Sometimes, the practical wisdom comes from parents who have been following this for a long time. We sincerely want to thank our parents for their help and encouragement. Some of them have silently guided us by living through these very principles. The knowledge dawns on novice practitioners like us only when we are mentally ready.

We are also grateful to our families for having helped us go through the marathon journey of food restrictions and slow lifestyle course-corrections. Special thanks to our spouses for having supported us with the special menu during the *Chaturmasa* months. We thank our friends, Vidya and Phani, for having edited the book and making major contributions to the structure and flow.

It is our verified & personal experience that *Chaturmasa* not only helps us appreciate food, and build discipline, it also helps us truly understand what it means to go hungry. Complying to the traditions of fasting according to *Sanatana Dharma,* we donate money and/or food to the needy.

Continuing the tradition of donation (*daanam*), we have decided to donate all proceeds from this book to help migrant children and their families who experience food scarcity and especially in these tough times of Covid. We are pledging support to donate all profits from this book to

Diya Ghar[1], an NGO in Bengaluru, India that is doing a yeoman service of supporting migrants and their families. For the last five years, Diya Ghar has been changing the lives of the migrant community in Bangalore by providing pre-school education for children of laborers in a nurturing environment. Along with foundational Montessori education, children are given two wholesome meals a day and safe transport from their settlements to school and back. So far, over 400 little ones have "graduated" from Diya Ghar and joined elementary schools in Bangalore or back in their villages.

In 2020 due to the constraints caused by Covid, Diya Ghar changed their model into a Community Centre. As of April 2021 they had 600 children in their preschool program and 1300 children receiving nutrition. Their goal is to reach 5,000 migrant children in Bengaluru.

We hope that readers who are inspired to practice *Ekadasi* and/or *Chaturmasa* after reading this book will recognize the positive impact they are having on the environment by not consuming more than what the body needs. The positive impact can also be quantified in dollars that can potentially be donated to those who face food scarcity, like the families that are supported by **Diya Ghar**. We firmly believe that this is the spirit of *daanam* as expounded in ancient *Sanatana Dharma* scriptures.

---

1   http://diyaghar.org

Why We Wrote This Book?

The year 2020 was a unique year in many ways. Life changed forever, with the Covid-19 pandemic shutting down the entire world, locking all of us in our homes. While it was extremely stressful and tragic for several, it was also an opportunity to go inside and discover our true self. It is said once we discover our true self, we see the entire transactional life as if it were a movie going on the screen, with the events, situations and happenings – neither good or bad – affecting us to the extent we let them.

Discovering who we truly are is an effort of many lifetimes for some. Yet, if one is focused and understands what the 'route map' the ancient scriptures prescribe, it could be completed within one lifetime, as emphatically declared by several spiritual *gurujis*.

Ancient scriptures like the *Gita, Upanishads, Yogasastra,* and mythological scriptures like the *Puranas* have a wealth of wisdom on the path we need to follow. While it is out of scope of this book to describe the path, it is clear that unless one has a strong, active, agile physical and mental constitution, it is difficult, nay impossible to understand who we truly are. Especially we need to prepare our minds, like a farmer who tills the soil, plants the seeds, waters the land, to receive the knowledge and live the wisdom in the scriptures.

Preparing our mind can be done in many ways and one of the first steps is to control and rein back our sensory inputs. Amongst the five sensory inputs, food is considered as one of the primary inputs that determine health – mental and physical. Hence, food and fasting have been given significance in ancient customs of India.

Eating healthy food, in limited quantities – as much as needed by the body, and regular fasting help the body build its immunity, improve life span and importantly, prepares the mind to understand complex subjects, like Self-knowledge. We can experience this intuitive fact in our daily lives as well. Think of how dull we feel after a heavy meal!

You probably heard of the Japanese scientist who won a Nobel Prize in 2016 for his discoveries of mechanisms of autophagy[2]. Dr. Yoshinori Ohsumi[3] discovered that there is a natural regulated mechanism of the cells to remove unnecessary or dysfunctional components. Fasting is known to trigger autophagy and this helps the body clean out unwanted, diseased cells.

Fasting is also considered as a way of getting in tune with nature and living in harmony with the changing lunar and solar cycles. Therefore every fortnight, we are expected to fast one day, and once every year, we are asked to change what we consume to tune ourselves to the changing seasons. Fortnightly fasting, known as *Ekadasi* helps us to attune to changes in nature due to lunar cycles and a complete diet change during the period known as *Chaturmasa* helps us to re-calibrate ourselves to changes in nature due to annual solar cycles.

While *Ekadasi* fasting is well-known and popular, which corresponds to the fortnightly fasting, the annual 'fasting' called *Chaturmasa* although popular in certain circles is not well-known in the modern days. The intuitive logic of *Chaturmasa* and the benefits make it an extremely potent way of building resilience as well as improve mental capacity and spiritual growth.

This book has been written for all those who may (or may not) have heard about *Chaturmasa* but needed more information on the practice, benefits and first hand experiences of practitioners. In the year 2020, five of

---

2   https://en.wikipedia.org/wiki/Autophagy

3   https://www.pbs.org/newshour/science/japanese-scientist-won-nobel-prize-cell-self-eating

us completed *Chaturmasa* and have extensively documented our learnings, experiences and relationship with food. The five editors of this book live in four different continents – Asia (India), Europe (UK), North America (USA) & Africa (Ghana) and have experienced immense benefits following the diet change regimen. We hope our experiences narrated in this book, will inspire you to experiment with *Chaturmasa*. Irrespective of where you live – tropical country or otherwise, we firmly believe the benefits of attuning oneself to annual solar cycles is immensely helpful for all.

A word of caution: Please always consult your doctor, and consider any pre-existing conditions that may need attention before embarking on any of the recommendations in this book. None of the practitioners are experts at offering medical advice that conforms either to Western medicine or Ayurveda. Our background is engineering and sciences and our objective is to share our transformation experiences to inspire others to live a healthy and happy lifestyle. We take no responsibility for any negative health outcomes by following any of the guidelines shared here. Neither would we ever claim any credit for any positive outcomes that you may have. It is the wisdom of the ancient sages and your earnest attitude that must be credited for the benefits.

Wellbeing Through Food & Discipline | The *Chaturmasa* Diaries is an attempt to inspire the reader to explore the path to their inner self through their relationship with food. Please note that we are careful to state that the exploration is *through* their relationship with food and are not saying that this exploration is *with* food..

Eat to Live or Live to Eat?

'To be or not to be' is the opening phrase of Hamlet, by William Shakespeare, contemplating on the choices facing him. Likewise, humanity is divided when it comes to answering the great question about food – **Eat to live or Live to Eat?**. While the majority will humorously dismiss this question, we cannot ignore the powerful, magnetic relationship we have with food. If one persists their inquiry, the seeming frivolous question will lead to deep philosophical answers reflecting human connection with food.

We clearly distinguish ourselves from animals. Evolution has given us more than the 'lower' beings – five sense organs (we have not yet discovered any other creature that has higher than five senses) and a highly evolved mind that is capable of connecting the dots from inputs coming through the five senses, recording it in memory, applying emotions and taking decisions. The sense of taste, amongst the five, is one of the powerful differentiators. Consequently, it is only natural that as time progressed, from paleolithic to the twenty-first century, humans experimented with food – from hunting to farming, from raw, uncooked to cooked and garnished.

We also differentiate ourselves through a higher sense of intelligence. Compared to animals and birds, we are endowed with higher intellectual faculties that make us superior. However, unless we uphold our responsibility as superior beings, we are the most deadly of all the living creatures in this universe. Despite the relative physical sizes of humans, the intellectual capacity in us makes us stronger than the elephants on land, the blue whales in the ocean or any creature of any size in between.

The human mind, working together with the various sense organs, especially the sense of taste, has redefined how we perceive food today.

The symbiotic relationship between food, the memory of food, recollection of the memories and their association with our emotional, physical well-being has become more important than the food itself.

Food is a major part of our societal fabric, making it an integral part of every get-together or social event. From times immemorial, food has served as a common denominator for bringing people together – sharing food is a common way to demonstrate that we care. A big part of expenses when one hosts major events like weddings is the quality of food one serves the guests. Likewise, it has become business culture to go out for lunch together with colleagues.

Food evokes emotions in us. It provides a feeling of comfort, happiness and contentment. Chocolates and sweet dishes are the recourse of many when one is stressed. While people in many parts of the world experience food shortage even today, there is no doubt that food has moved beyond the 'necessity/need' category. It has become a 'want' for us. Food now is a primal desire and source of enjoyment, perhaps even higher on the priority list than sex.

Food as Medicine or Medicine as Food?

According to *Taittiriya* Upanishad, one of the principal *Upanishads*, which explains how *Brahman* or the Supreme Soul in every being can be realized, using a technique known as *pancha kosa viveka*, literally translated as 'knowledge of the five sheaths', the definition of 'food' (*annam* in *Samskritam)* is **'that which beings eat and which eats beings'**.

Here below is an excerpt from the *Upanishad*[4]:

अन्नाद्वै प्रजा: प्रजायन्ते । या: काश्च पृथिवीं श्रिता: ।
अथो अन्नेनैव जीवन्ति । अथैनदपि यन्त्यन्तत: ।
अन्नं हि भूतानां ज्येष्ठम् । तस्मात् सर्वौषधमुच्यते ।
सर्वं वै ते ऽन्नमाप्नुवन्ति । ये ऽन्नं ब्रह्मोपासते ।
अन्नं हि भूतानां ज्येष्ठम् । तस्मात् सर्वौषधमुच्यते ।
अन्नाद् भूतानि जायन्ते । जातान्यन्नेन वर्धन्ते ।
अद्यतेऽत्ति च भूतानि । तस्मादन्नं तदुच्यत इति ॥ १ ॥

annadvai prajah prajayante, yah kasca prthivigmsritah,
atho annenaiva jivanti, athainadapi yantyantatah,
annagmhi bhutanam jyestham, tasmatsarvausadhamucyate,
sarvam vai te'nnamapnuvanti, ye'nnam brahmopasate,
annagm hi bhutanam jyestham, tasmatsarvausadhamucyate,
annadbhutani jayante, jatanyannena vardhante,
adyate'tti ca bhutani, tasmadannam taducyata iti ॥ 1 ॥

All beings that exist on earth are born of food. They, thereafter, live by food; again, they ultimately go back to it and merge to become food, So, verily, food is the eldest of all the creatures. On that ground it is called the medicament for all. Those who meditate on Brahman as food, indeed obtain all food, from food all beings are born, having been born, they grow by (consuming) food. Food is that which is eaten by the beings and also that which in the end eats them; therefore, food is called annam. [II – II – 1]

It may sound like a strange definition of food, but it is true at multiple levels.

Here is a very high level, simplistic, intuitive reason for such a definition: Whatever food living beings eat, nourishes them and it becomes part of them. When the beings die, their body becomes food for someone else – either directly or indirectly.

4　Page 18 of the document in https://vedantastudents.com/wp-content/uploads/2018/10/05-Taittriya-Upanishad-Summary.pdf

Also, here is another insight that we observe in our life.

What happens when we overeat? Prolonged overeating results in obesity and several diseases like cardiovascular, lower body flexibility and breathing problems. Over time, these problems will begin to 'consume' us, giving rise to health issues and even death. In 2005, the World Health Organization (WHO) estimated that 61 per cent of all deaths -- 35 million -- and 49 per cent of the global burden of disease were attributable to chronic 'lifestyle' diseases. By 2030, the proportion of total global deaths due to chronic diseases is expected to increase to 70 per cent and the global burden of disease to 56 per cent. Lifestyle diseases share risk factors similar to prolonged exposure to three modifiable lifestyle behaviors -- smoking, unhealthy diet, and physical inactivity -- and result in the development of chronic diseases, specifically heart disease, stroke, diabetes, obesity, metabolic syndrome, chronic obstructive pulmonary disease, and some types of cancer.[5]

Here again is a third insight which is again intuitive.

If we eat/drink the wrong type of food, for example, sustained alcoholic drinking or consuming food that is stale, impure/contaminated, we could end up with health issues. The health issues in turn will 'consume' us.

So, what happens to an individual that consumes food indiscriminately, either more than what is required for the body, or the wrong types of food than what the body needs?

Chances are the person will fall sick sooner or later. Once we fall sick, the first thing the doctors will restrict is the diet. And, unfortunately, if the sickness is severe, we will end up consuming a lot of medication – as if we were 'replacing' food.

It is our choice: Either we consume food as medicine or consume medicine as food.

---

5   https://www.un.org/en/chronicle/article/lifestyle-diseases-economic-burden-health-services

We would prefer the first choice. Reverence to food we eat has to become a habit – because it is a symbiotic relationship between food and the consumer. Like one of the spiritual gurus says, the bread you ate for breakfast or the apple for dinner becomes some part of your body. Quality of inputs is important. So, consume only what the body needs.

Bhagavan Sri Krishna also explains to *Arjuna* in *sloka 17* of Chapter 6[6] that a moderate eating habit is an essential spiritual practice. He further explains in Chapter 17, *slokas* 8,9,10[7] as to what type of food a person should eat or not eat.

For an excellent overview on how ancient scriptures view 'food', please refer to this article by Divine Life Society, *Upanishads* on Food[8].

---

6   *Sloka* 17 Chapter 6 of *Gita* https://www.holy-bhagavad-gita.org/chapter/6/verse/17

7   *Sloka 8 of Chapter 17 of Gita* on Food: https://www.holy-bhagavad-gita.org/chapter/17/verse/8

8   https://www.sivanandaonline.org/public_html/?cmd=displaysection§ion_id=771&parent=762&format=html

The New Age of Diet Plans

New year. New beginnings. New hopes. We eagerly make resolutions to stay fit, be healthy, workout more or reduce weight.

Unfailingly every year, *#weight* and *#diets* are two top search topics on Google, that see an increasing trend and continue to be of interest all year around for people worldwide. Take a look at the following comparison chart[9], from Google Trends and you will notice a sustained interest since 2004!

With the high level of interest in healthy living, different time-tested, proven diets prop up time and again, finding their niche, offering benefits of health, weight loss, muscle tone, resistance to diseases and truly creating healthy lifestyle changes.

In 2018, Forbes published an article, on top six asked-about diets that have piqued people's curiosity with their promise to deliver real results. *#Keto, #Paleo, #Alkaline, #Whole 30, #Intermittent Fasting, #Carb Cycling* are not mere words for those in their pursuit of health, weight loss and looking & being fit.

These diets have the possibility of changing our lives, and in fact, several people claim so. A look at the Reddit, will justify this with the **top 3 being Keto, Intermittent Fasting & Paleo**. Keto community is 873,000 people strong, followed by Intermittent Fasting of 177,000 people and Paleo at 125,000 people.

---

9   https://trends.google.com/trends/explore?q=diet,weight

Closer home, within our circle of reach, the interest in fitness & health and discussions on different dietary techniques is quite high. Thanks to Whatsapp groups between family, friends it is not uncommon to encourage each other on a 3 day juicing diet, 10 day liquid diet, intermittent fasting, high protein diet, 10 day Ayurvedic detox diet or the vegan diet.

We also have started noticing companies like Weight Watchers[10], Noom[11] offering diet plans, recipes and even portion controlled foods. It has created a new industry in itself.

Our conclusion is that ALL these diet plans work.

Any diet where we go back to the basics will surely work wonders. Cutting out processed, and unhealthy food, reducing quantity intake can result in dramatic changes which we will be happy about. While we subscribe to the view that we should follow what would work for us, it is best to review our goals once a while. All the diets that are mentioned in the Forbes article focus mostly on physical health benefits. However, it is absolutely critical to ask and re-evaluate our goal. If our goal orientation is physical health only, we can pick any of the top asked-about diets and reap the benefits.

Unfortunately, choosing physical health benefits alone is a myopic view, which forces us to think narrowly about the benefits. A tunnel-vision goal is essential at times, but we feel that perhaps, this is a result of over emphasis on looking good and being physically fit, slim & attractive. This has been an outcome of society having been fed with misinformation about what physical beauty is all about. Who decides what is attractive and what is ugly? It is the notion in the heads of product managers, advertisers, perhaps even poets and authors who have described physical beauty in their words and the entire society seems to have accepted certain arbitrary characteristics as pinnacle of physical beauty. And, why do we succumb to the societal notions of beauty to the extent that models end

---

10 https://www.weightwatchers.com/us/
11 https://www.noom.com

up being anorexic? Why isn't fat (or 'being rounded') beautiful? While we acknowledge that our bodies are very important, in the Eastern tradition, our physical body is considered just one aspect of ourselves. Numerous scientific studies have proven what Eastern traditions have long proclaimed for 5000 years, that there is a mind-body connection and we are much more than the physical body.

Nobody denies this fact, yet we know so little about what constitutes a human being beyond the physical body. A quick look at the modern medicine system indicates that the doctors specialize in different parts of the human body, and are adept at treating humans for their physical illness, but very few address the psychological and emotional illnesses. Yet, none of us can deny that we don't ever feel mentally unwell. Neither can we deny that we don't experience ourselves beyond the physical.

What if our goal was to nourish our entire body – the physical & the non-physical? What diet would work well for such a goal?

The Ancient Eastern Practices

Spiritual Context

Unlike Western medicine, in yogic tradition a human being is modeled as multiple 'bodies' layered together. In fact, the Eastern spiritual science models it as 'five sheaths'[12] – *pancha kosa* model of a human.

- First, is the physical body, built with muscles, bones, blood that is nourished by food we eat. It is what we all perceive, touch & feel.

- The subtle body has three components:

    - physiological (energy/*pranic*) body, emotional (*manah*) body, and intellectual (*buddhih*) body.

- Finally we have the causal (*kaarana*) body, which has no equivalent in modern science as yet.

Energy body controls the five basic human body processes of respiration, digestion, elimination, circulation & involuntary processes like hiccups. Mind is unseen, yet the most powerful entity we all experience, consisting of memory, emotions, intellect and 'ego'. Memory, emotions and 'ego' can be considerd as emotional body. Intellectual body is the decision making, rational faculty.

Very little research is being done today in the Western world to understand what types of foods we should eat to nourish the entire human being – who is composed of five layered bodies as described above.

---

12 For details on five sheath model, please refer to https://www.swami-krishnananda. org/panchadasi/pan_14.html

However, the yogic & Ayurvedic tradition from the East has several recommendations. These recommendations, when followed are diets that would nourish the physical body and importantly, the subtle body as well. Moreover, eating and fasting are two sides of the same coin. They go hand in hand. Who can say they have experienced happiness unless they have experienced what is sadness and vice-versa?

Surprisingly, East's yogic recommendations have little to do with carbohydrates, proteins, fats, minerals but more in terms of the **qualitative content** of food (*gunas)* we eat.

It is interesting to note the claim that the subtle body is nourished by the subtle elements in the food we consume, while the gross physical body is nourished by the gross elements. Different foods that we eat, beyond the all familiar nutritional dietary value, are also known to have different quality or virtue (*'guna'*[13], in *Samskritam,* which is a difficult word to translate in English). All foods have one of three qualities (three *gunas)* – *sattva, rajas, tamas* (again, difficult words to translate in English). Yogic tradition claims that foods with these qualities contribute to different aspects of our holistic health.

- *Sattvic* foods increase our perceptive (knowledge, learnability, memory) abilities

- *Rajasic* foods increase our activity levels (physical & mental work) and

- *Tamasic* foods increase our laziness (sleep, sloth, boredom) qualities

So, in addition to asking how many proteins, carbohydrates, fats & minerals our food has, we should also ask if they are *sattvic, rajasic* or *tamasic* foods. We provide a list of foods categorized by their *gunas* later on in this book as a reference.

---

13 For an overview of *guna* concept in general, please refer to https://www.sivanandaonline.org/public_html/?cmd=displaysection§ion_id=878

It is important to note that there are five senses that feed our subtle body (consisting of emotional mind, intellect, memory) and food is one of them, but an important one. It is equally important to exercise restraint on the other senses as well. From this point of view, it helps to view food as one of the 'inputs' to the body, along with other four – auditory (through ears), sight (through eyes), tactile (through skin) and olfactory (through nose). These nourish the subtle body as well. No wonder that one feels hungry when one smells amazing food even before seeing or tasting it.

It is important to recognize the reasons why we are covering the five sheath model in so much detail. What use is the muscles we develop if we have poor digestion or circulation or evacuation processes within our body? What use is our physical health if we struggle with mental health issues? Therefore, managing subtle body efficiently is key and a means to automatically managing our physical body. Science has several studies that have documented the ill-effects of stress, negative emotions, thoughts on our body and has linked lifestyle diseases as psycho somatic.

There is another deeper spiritual reason for managing the subtle body well. It is the subtle body that becomes most important tool/instrument (*karanam*) towards a human being's ultimate goal and search for eternal happiness/bliss. Even without reading any scriptures, it is clear that all beings search for more happiness (*sukha*)and want to reduce as much unhappiness/pain (*dukhah*). So, even arguing logically, we all are in an quest for eternal happiness/bliss. In this quest, a subtle body is said to last several lifetimes compared to a physical body that perishes at death. According to *Sanatana Dharma*'s theory of reincarnation[14], a being sheds its physical body upon death while the subtle body (*sukshma sharira*) travels to find another suitable body till such time the embodied soul has realized *Brahman,* the Universal Soul, by gaining knowledge of its true Self and staying in that knowledge[15].

---

14 *Sloka* 22 of Chapter 2 in *Bhagavad Gita* states that just as a person sheds worn-out garments and wears new ones, likewise, at the time of death, the subtle body casts off its worn-out body and enters a new one.

15 This is also known as *moksha*, liberation from all sorts of problems, limitations, fears, insecurities one experiences in transactional life.

Human birth is considered a privilege and provides an opportunity to get out of the misery of the near-perennial life-birth-death cycle of a transmigratory soul. This is known as *moksha* or complete mental freedom from any sort of limitations we experience – of space, time, position, power, objects or people. While it may not be the goal of several people to attain the eternal freedom that the scriptures proclaim as our very birthright, it is surely a goal of all to live a healthy, disease free life.

In either case, we need to develop holistic health – physical and importantly subtle body health to reach the chosen goal. Developing holistic health is a matter of choice and discipline, which only humans are capable of exhibiting among all species in this creation.

While there are four similarities between an animal and a human birth – eat, sleep, procreate and exhibit fear, the biggest differentiator is our ability to exhibit free-will and control our senses. According to several scriptures[16], controlling our sense organs is one of the key prerequisites for healthy living – at a physical and emotional level.

Any sort of voluntary sense control, including delayed gratification – a word so commonly used in the modern investment/consumerism context, is known as *tapah*. The *Sanskritam* word, *tapah* literally means 'to turn the heat on'. *Tapah* essentially 'burns' something by the heat it generates in the body at physical and mental level and in turn this heat reduces the impact of our deep driven desires, tendencies, cravings and makes us more calmer, perceptive and joyous. Think of *tapah* similar to the intense discipline of a

---

16   *Sloka 17 of* Chapter 2 in *Bhagavad Gita* states: But those who are temperate in eating and recreation, balanced in work, and regulated in sleep, can mitigate all sorrows by practicing Yoga. There are other references to control of food intake, sensory control in several other scriptures like *Yoga Sutras* by *Maharshi Patanjali* and *Hatha Yoga Pradipika*

    Sloka 5 of Chapter 18 in *Bhagavad Gita* states: Work (activity) in the spirit of sacrifice (selflessness/or service to others – *seva)*, donations/gifts given of our wealth, knowledge and time, and austerities should not be relinquished, but should indeed be performed for these help the individual to become more aligned with their true Self by bringing clarity and focus to their minds ('sanctifying').

sportsman who wants to win Olympic gold. *Tapah* is also a precondition to reducing our innate fickle minded nature, enabling us to focus on any chosen subject. In another classical scriptural text called *Sadhana Chatushtaya*[17] *tapah* is also referred to as *damah*, sense control. It is one of the four folded essential qualifications under the sub-category, *shama-dama-adi*. It is said that unless one exhibits sensory control, especially in their eating habits it is difficult to understand the subtle concepts of Universal Soul (*Brahman*), Individual Soul (*Atma*), Ego-sense (*Ahamkara*), and subtle body (*sukshma sharira*, consisting of physiological, emotional, intellectual and potential capabilities of a human being). This is because, the the quality of food, as determined by its *gunas* has a direct impact on our subtle body as well and has a potential to make us receptive, digressive or lazy. There are several ways these *gunas* manifest in food – the type of food we eat, the quantity we consume are two major factors that we will discuss more in this book.

Yogic traditions recommend us to take a holistic view of who we are – not just viewing physical health, redefine our goal and then choose the right diet plan. It is easy to dismiss the simplicity of this approach at our own loss. Just as Steve Jobs hid the complexity of technology in an iPhone and presented to the world in terms of the simple & intuitive user experience, the yogic tradition hides the complexities and presents few simple plans for us to follow.

In our research as practitioners[18] and, from the multitude of diet plans from the yogic tradition, we would recommend the following two – *Ekadasi* and *Chaturmasa*. Strictly speaking, these two are not 'diets' in the conventional sense of the usage of the word, 'diet plan' and we will explain this concept a bit in future chapters. One can ease into these plans very smoothly and they easily and quickly integrate into one's life. They are not mutually exclusive but complement each other.

---

17 Refer to *Sadhana Chatushtaya Sampatthi here, https://www.swami-krishnananda.org/spiritual.aspiration/aspiration_6.html*

18 One of the editors of this booklet is a yoga & meditation coach for decades

Ekadasi

The diet plan in this is simple, with an ultimate goal of not eating or drinking for a day every fortnight! One does not eat or drink anything after sunset the previous day, till sunrise of the following day, roughly resting the body for 36 hours in all.[19] In the beginning, it may appear like a "starving" day, however as one practices with patience and determination, the body and mind self-regulates and longs for the "fasting" day. Several naturopathy homes that treat chronic diseases use fasting as one of the mechanisms to revive the body's innate ability to repair itself.

The *Samskritam* word *Eka-dasi* consisting of the words, *eka & dasi* literally means eleventh day. Typically, this is the eleventh day after a full moon or new moon. The scriptures recommend us to fast on this particular day to neutralize the effect of planetary positions, especially of the moon. Given that the human body has over 75% water content, it is not incomprehensible that our body is influenced by the lunar cycles as much as the tides in the ocean are. While it is recommended to fast on these two specific days every month, we would not worry too much about the specificity as long as we stick to fasting once every fortnight.

In the final stages of this plan, we aim to not eat or drink anything at all. However, not everybody will be physically & mentally prepared to do this. Just as anything requires gradual, consistent practice, this aim can easily become a lifestyle in about six months. We can start by eating healthy on the chosen day including only fruits, nuts & milk in as much quantity as your body needs (and we want to emphasize – it is needs, **not** wants!). Over time, reduce the quantity and eat only when one is hungry (sorry, no munching!). Over many fortnights, one can gradually reduce the quantity and completely be on water (or an occasional fruit).

The logic behind this simple fasting can look counter-intuitive for the followers of popular diet plans that we summarized earlier. But, rest

---

19 To clarify this, if the fasting 'day' is a Monday, then you will not eat anything from Sunday evening sunset till Tuesday morning sunrise.

assured that millions in the East follow this traditional fortnightly fasting even today, and the practice is prevalent from time immemorial[20].

When we fast, we rest our digestive system. When it is rested, different organs and body processes need to do less work. Then the body's innate ability turns its attention to detoxify itself and eliminate waste and toxins from the body. This improves our immune system and helps ward off illnesses. There are several research papers being published about the connection fasting has on incurable diseases like cancer. In one study[21], it is said that fasting or fasting-mimicking diets (FMDs) generate environments that can reduce the capability of cancer cells to adapt and survive as well as increase resistance to chemotherapy in normal but not cancer cells and promote regeneration in normal tissues. In fact, it is common advice to starve a fever, letting the body rest completely and recover. With the stomach being empty, the blood flow increases towards the brain. This nourishes the brain, making our perception and reflexes sharper, improving memory, better judgement and calmness. Moreover, it is our common experience that there are more deaths and diseases caused by overeating[22], than by abstaining from food.

It is also said that avoiding certain food items like onion, garlic, green chilies, frozen food, food that has been cooked & kept either in the fridge or in the open for more than 12 hours, all types of meats, poultry, seafood improves the quality of our perception and aids in acquiring & retaining knowledge. Avoiding such food helps reduce the *tamasic* & *rajasic* quality of the food. We recognize that in the Western world, certain foods may be difficult to let go and we propose the practitioner modify their food based on the guidelines provided later in the book on the *gunas* of these foods.

---

20 There are scriptural references in abundance about the benefits of *Ekadasi* fasting.

21 https://www.ncbi.nlm.nih.gov/pmc/articles/PMC6938162/

22 We are qualifying this statement to include deaths that are caused by lifestyle diseases like heart attacks, diabetes. All these can be managed well through lifestyle changes, especially with food. We also refer you to the article by United Nations which we referenced earlier on in the book regarding chronic/lifestyle diseases.

Chaturmasa

Strictly by the English definition of 'fasting' we cannot consider *Chaturmasa* as fasting. It is more of a 'diet plan' to suit the changing seasons. However, we will use the word 'seasonal fasting' when we refer to *Chaturmasa.*

The diet plan in this is to eat foods in limited quantities and within certain 'allowed' categories of foods. Unlike *ekadasi,* where we are asked to abstain from eating/drinking completely, here the restrictions are on what we can eat and when, and these are tuned to the changing seasons. The spiritual references to *Chaturmasa* is in most of the *puranas*[23]. Everybody above sixteen years of age is encouraged, without exception, to follow this practice.

The seasonal fasting is applicable and relevant especially for people living in tropical countries, where major seasonal changes occur during the last week of July to the last week in November. One might wonder how convincing is this really for other geographical regions where seasons are different and food supply chains are different? The editors of this book live in four continents – Africa, Asia, Europe and North America and have experienced similar benefits and, we are of the opinion that this may be universally applicable.

---

23 Puranas, https://en.wikipedia.org/wiki/Puranas are stories that have been part of *Sanatana Dharma* tradition where the esoteric spiritual concepts were re-told in a tangible, easy-to-imbibe form. For example, a story that depicts a lion-man form of the Supreme soul, *Narasimha avatara.* While the story itself is very simple, the symbolic significance of why the form of a lion-man is very deep. Just as a 'head' is the leader of the rest of the body, a lion is the leader in the jungle. Humans have both these qualities within us – to lead others and to be led. This symbolism of man-lion is to show us that the leader is within us (the Supreme Soul or *Atma,* or even conscience – if one prefers this word) and the one led is also within us – our ego, intellect, emotional mind (in short, our subtle body).

There are also several studies[24] being done to correlate the rise of pathogens, diseases and food outbreaks to the seasons. However, we are convinced of the benefits that this plan will provide to practitioners living in any part of the world. We base this on the fundamental fact that the Eastern traditions measure the value of food very differently based on the 'quality' as represented by its *gunas*, freshness and less about the calorific or nutritional value as presented in the West. Not consuming foods that have *tamasic guna* in them is the simplest way to improve health – physical and mental, irrespective of where one lives.

Yogic tradition asks us to avoid certain types of food in these four months.

- With the onset of rains in July-August, vegetables especially greens come with the danger of insects & worms causing health issues if we consume them.

- August-September-October, usually being the time when pregnant cows are in their final leg before delivering the calves, the milk (and also its derivatives, by-products) is considered to be unhealthy for human consumption. Initially, we avoid yoghurt and later milk for a month each.

- Finally in October-November months, with the onset of cold weather, vegetables grown below the ground are considered to increase the body heat & provide the right nutrients to the body while we are asked to avoid lentils & legumes.

With the guidelines for quality of food described above, we discuss quantity of food consumed. As in fortnightly fasting, our goal is to reduce the quantity of food intake, but not completely. We have to find an optimum

---

24 An article that explains how human body adapts to seasons concluding with the known fact that higher is related to lower light levels during fall seasons and lower depression during the spring months: https://www.scientificamerican.com/article/to-every-pathogen-there-is-a-season/

Here is another publication, https://www.nature.com/articles/s41598-020-74435-9

level of intake that our body needs (not wants!). Think of this as running a marathon, than a hundred meter dash. Just as the training & practice are different for running both these races, we follow different techniques for seasonal fasting.

How do we know if we are eating adequate quantity of food?

Yogic tradition once again saves the day by asking us to eat half our stomach with solids, quarter with water and leave the remaining space for digestive processes to work on. We can experiment and arrive at optimal levels based on trial and error method. There are certain 'measures' provided as well in this book to redue the time taken to experiment and we recommend you to consider those measures as well.

The tradition also recommends us to eat only vegetarian food, and avoid meat, poultry and seafood. Again, in the Western world, this may be difficult to follow. Our recommendation is to first focus on reducing the quantity of food intake and eat half stomach full, during these four months. Over time, we can switch to a plant-based food (while eliminating onion, garlic and green chilies) during these four months.

We would recommend you to try *Chaturmasa* fasting after completing six months of fortnightly fasting and preparing your body and mind adequately to deepen and nourish your body & mind. There is no harm in trying *Chaturmasa* independently as well for those who have strong willpower and determination.

Finally a word about the timing of *Chaturmasa:* Unlike dates in the Gregorian calendar, the calendar system that we use to calculate the start and end of *Chaturmasa* are based on the planetary positions and these vary from year to year. It is also important to remember that once in four years, an extra month is used as an adjustment (similar to the concept of leap year) and we fast for five months instead of four months.

Other Fasting References

While the Indian culture enjoys and celebrates food, fasting is very common during most festivals. One will also notice that fasting is more or less 'prescribed' by almost all religions – *Ramadan* (Muslims), Lent (Christians), *Paryushan* (Jains) are some of the popular fasting festivals of a few religions. Interestingly, *Paryushan* is synchronized with *Chaturmasa*.

Scriptural Context of *Chaturmasa*

We observe that the life span of different species in this world are different. A human lives for approximately 80 years while a tortoise lives for over 200 whereas a firefly may live for a day or a few days. Beyond the observable, scriptures state that there are celestial beings, known as *devas*[25], who have different life spans. For the atheists, we can think of these celestial beings as different natural energy principles, like space, air, fire, water, earth, time, rain, wealth, knowledge, love, valor, protection, procreation, destruction etc. It is said that these natural principles rest in a 'form' of *deva*, and are deified and worshipped in that form. Explaining the concept of *devas* beyond this is out of scope of this book and we refer you to read several scriptures starting with *Mahabharata* or *Ramayana* – the two great epics from India which cover these in many details, before graduating to read *Puranas*. The idols that we see in temples are a representative indication of the energy principle behind.

A day in the celestial world is equal to one year of humans. Just as human beings' innate capabilities wax and wane during the day, the strength of these divine energy principles waxes and wanes during their day time. For example, we see that most of us are active during the day time, when the sun is shining and go off to sleep and rest during night. And when we are asleep, there is a certain period of our sleep corresponding to 'light' sleep and another period to 'deep' sleep. Usually, the light sleep occurs within the first hour of us lying down and the last hour before we wake up,

---

25 The word *deva* literally means, who shines on their own – basically to indicate that they are beings whose bodies are not like the forms found in this earth, but of a different body that is luminous with knowledge (not to be mistaken for 'light')

and in between is when we find ourselves sleeping soundly without a care in this world.

To understand how we can apply the concept of 'deep' sleep to the celestial beings, we have to understand a bit about astronomy as viewed by Indian astrological science. Astronomers have noticed a 'northwardly apparent movement of sun, around the winter solstice time (last week of December) till summer solstice time (last week of June). The northward movement starts from the Tropic of Capricorn and ends at the Tropic of Cancer. The northward movement is known as *Uttarayana*[26] (*Uttara* – north; *ayana* – path) and the southward movement known as *Dakshinayana* (*Dakshina* – south).

Like our sleep pattern, the middle four months between summer solstice and winter solstice is considered as the period of 'deep sleep' for the celestials, so there is no positive support for our earthly activities. What it means is that the energy principles in the universe have lower energy levels during these four months. Nature therefore does not support with tail-wind to beings living on earth to conduct their activities. Therefore, if a being has to live in harmony with these natural principles, the food and other habits also need to be modified to suit the environmental conditions during that time. Interestingly, these four months of each year are considered inauspicious for undertaking any sort of major initiative, like wedding, travel etc.

With this insight into how the cosmos functions and knowledge of advanced science of astrology, our ancient *rishis*[27] divined the concept of

---

26 http://isatsang.blogspot.com/2016/01/significance-of-ayanas-dakshinayana-and.html

27 A *rishi* is a sage, who has the ability to understand the mysteries of the universe in exactly the way it is and guides the rest of the lesser mortals with easy to follow principles. For example, Sage Viswamitra gave us a principle to meditate on the divine energy of the sun, known as *Gayatri Mantra*. The energy of the sun, which nourishes the plants, invigorates life on this planet is 'embodied' in that *manta*, or chant and it is believed by millions that chanting *Gayatri Mantra* bestows health, better eyesight (as Sun is the presiding deity of eyes!) and a sharp intellect.

Chaturmasa prescribing what foods are conducive to eat, what activities can be done or to be avoided during this period. In a nutshell, if we would like to understand this in modern terms, it is similar to a plan with do's & don'ts to sail taking advantage of the tides in the sea. Or, using the tailwinds to fly faster in the sky. It is finding harmony with nature.

To satisfy the reader's curiosity, we recommend you to read an overview from a deeper scriptural reference perspective, from the following two sites:

https://resanskrit.com/what-is-chaturmas-Ekadasi/

https://en.wikipedia.org/wiki/Chaturmas

How We Felt at Finish Line

In this chapter, we provide you the final summary of how each of the five participants felt completing *Chaturmasa* in 2020. In the following chapter, monthly 'intermediate' summaries are presented to give the reader an experience of the progress each participant was making every month. We would encourage you to read these two chapters together.

Journey to Discover, Who Am I?

With the grace of *Daivam*[28], I completed my first *Chaturmasa*, thanks to the persistent pitch of one of us who had been practicing this for several years, constant encouragement from my *co-Chaturmasa* friends and my wife's patience with the demands of my *sankalp*[29]!

This blog captures my experiences over 5 months (this year was an extra month) together with some reflections. I hope it will be helpful for those who wish to do this in the years ahead.

Why *Chaturmasa?*

I asked myself this question before *Chaturmasa* and also researched the same, but candidly, I could not find any clear answers. I was therefore hesitant, while the mind saw some rationale behind this time-tested observance (it marks the period of abstinence during the period our Gods are resting per *Vedic* timeline), the intellect was not entirely convinced of

---

28 The Divine

29 *Sankalp* is a *Samskritam* word for a firm resolution – something that one would stick to because it is important. https://en.wikipedia.org/wiki/Sankalpa

its benefits. It felt like a good test of will-power but there were self-doubts that the *sankalp* might not sustain once the initial excitement wore off.

Having weighed it all up and with the motivation of my friends, I decided to give it a go, hoping it would be an exercise in self-control. Subconsciously, there was a latent desire to get rid of some of the stubborn pounds, which (most) middle-aged folks like me seem to accumulate and struggle with to be rid of.

I progressively began to appreciate the meaning of *Chaturmasa* while experiencing it. It's all about following a *Sattva* life-style – eating right (vegetarian), moderating eating habits, regular sleep cycle, doing *yogasanas* & breathing exercises, spiritual thoughts, reduced screen time, seeking blessings from elders, austerity, charity, to mention a few.

Chaturmasa is less about food and more about developing a contemplative mind, moderating desires and moving towards *Santosham* (contentment). It involves putting into practice the tenets of *Sadhana Chatushtaya Sampatti* or the four-fold qualifications for pursuing spiritual growth, in particular *Samaha* (mind control), *Damaha* (sense control), *Titiksha* (forbearance) & *Vairagya* (dispassion).

Reliving the Experience

To begin with, the emphasis was primarily on food, there was a lot of early excitement and chatter around what to eat and recipes, with several pictures of amazing dishes being shared! Eating only two meals a day with portion control was hard and we sought refuge in our favourites, for me the mango season early on was such a saviour! I ended up indulging in excessive healthy snacking (fruits and nuts) to satisfy my hunger pangs, particularly after dinner. However, by the end of July, we had settled into a cadence, increasingly comfortable with eating less than we usually did while enduring some difficult days. Old snacking habits die hard!

Over time, food increasingly became less important as the overall spiritual quotient improved. I regularly listened to Vedantic discourses – I managed to learn *NirvanaShatakam*[30], *PratahSmaranam Stotram*[31] and the *Shanti Mantra*[32], all very powerful and meaningful. It has since become a habit and I now chant them every day.

Initially, I felt a bit disoriented and concerned about looking and/or feeling weak. However, those moments of self-doubt came and went and we smoothly transitioned from 'no-veggies' to 'no-yogurt' to 'no-milk' to 'no-seeds' diet during the five months. The final month though was quite a slog – with no fruits (except bananas & dates), no above-ground vegetables or lentils. I sensed a lack of balance in my diet and despite a lot of milk products, my body felt bloated. I did not particularly enjoy it but persisted nevertheless, it was a useful reminder that sometimes we have to do things which we may not necessarily like.

Interestingly, I was able to join my family on the dining table, while they ate a more appetizing meal or enjoyed a birthday spread and I was completely fine with it. My pre-*Chaturmasa* motto was 'live to eat' but I now appreciate that we eat to live and that 'food is an instrument and not an end in itself'.

Ekadasi fasting was another wonderful experience, it comes twice a month per the lunar calendar, on the 11th day after the new-moon and full-moon days and is usually done without eating or drinking anything and by turning our awareness inwards. I was unsure if I could endure that level of discipline & self-control, but I progressively moved from eating one meal (lest I got a headache) to only fruits to drinking only warm water to

---

30 https://www.cse.iitb.ac.in/~siva/nirvana.pdf Adi Sankaracharya, who wrote this *sloka*, summarizes the entire knowledge that we need to truly learn. Watch this YouTube video here for a rendering of the *sloka* along with its deeper meaning: https://youtu.be/-V5JkDyk2g0

31 https://www.kamakoti.org/shlokas/kshlok2.htm. Even this *sloka* was written by Sri. Adi Sankaracharya

32 Every *Veda* has a *shanti mantra* – a rendering seeking peace in the macro, micro environments and also within ourselves. Check this link for a few, https://timesofindia. indiatimes.com/religion/mantras-chants/bring-peace-home-with-the-shanti-mantra/ articleshow/75429866.cms

eventually not even drinking water – *Nirjala* – on *Dev-Utthana Ekadasi*[33] (the day Gods wake up) to complete the *sankalp*! It gives the body much needed rest and contrary to my expectation, I actually felt quite energetic the next morning. However, I would advise reduced physical activity during the fast to avoid losing excessive body salts. I also realized that the two-meals regime allows for a 14–15 hour intermittent fasting every day, ensuring all the food is fully digested.

I also experimented with a humbling experience of seeking forgiveness from some folks I may have hurt, intentionally or otherwise during the Jain holy week of *Paryushan*. I fasted during *Navratri* as well as on *Krishna Ashtami* and enjoyed *Diwali* festivities with milk based sweets, given the restrictions! [34]

I have to highlight that I had the good fortune of doing *Chaturmasa* together with a few similarly inclined and super enthusiastic, *co-Chaturmasa* friends, which kept me going and made my experience really enjoyable. We learnt from each other on our WhatsApp group and through regular calls. I would not have been able to complete the *sankalp* without their constant encouragement, guidance and support as I dealt with bouts of self-doubts or an occasional frustrating day.

What went well?

As mentioned above, this has been a 'lifestyle changing' experience for me. I am writing this a week after finishing *Chaturmasa* but I am continuing with a similar regimen, of course without undue restrictions and I have not felt any urge to default back to my earlier routine.

---

33 https://en.wikipedia.org/wiki/Prabodhini_Ekadashi

34 *Navratri, Krishna-Ashtami* and *Diwali* are popular festivals in India which are celebrated with fasting in some circles and feasting in others.

At a personal level, I regularly did *yoga asanas, pranayama* and *dhyana*[35] besides walking (and running) every single day (as an aside, I completed 500 consecutive days of *pranayama* on Nov 27th). Having averaged 15k steps/11km a day, I lost 7kgs, I am now at 67kg (though I expect to pull it back up a little bit) and I am now able to do asanas that I could not even contemplate earlier as my flexibility increased. I have been regularly listening to a variety of scriptural discourses by Swami Sarvapriyananada[36], Swami Parmarthmananda[37] and others, which nicely complements the *Gita* sessions I participate in every Sunday together with some of my friends (all are collectively my Gurus).

To satiate my food cravings, healthy snacking including fruits, buttermilk and healthy nuts worked quite well. *Ekadasi* fasts were a great way to detox regularly. I am pleased that regular yoga coupled with *Sattva* food habits have helped reduce the frequency as well as intensity & recovery of my painful chronic lower backaches. During the entire *Chaturmasa* period, it happened just once as against every month earlier. I am an 'impatient' Type 1 personality, but I sense that I am now somewhat calmer and also more accepting of different viewpoints – *Anekantavaad*[38] – on topics where I have a different viewpoint.

What could I have done better?

One of my goals has been *Samaha* or mind control, but I have struggled to focus my monkey mind. I am trying different meditation techniques like *Japa*, soft chanting, or just reciting a prayer, and I shall work on it over the next several months.

---

35 We can connect back these three terms – *yogasanas, pranayama & dhyana* to the *pancha-kosha* model of a human being. *Yogasanas* predominantly help at the physical body levels through the various postures. *Pranayama* helps the subtle body – the physiological body controlling the inner processes. Finally, *dhyana*, also known commonly, yet incorrectly as meditation, helps in concentration, focus and clarity.

36 https://www.vedantany.org/resident-swamis/

37 https://arshavidya.org/tribute-by-swami-paramarthananda/

38 https://en.wikipedia.org/wiki/Anekantavada

I was hoping to listen to Swami Sarvapriyananda's lecture series on *Aparokshanubhuti*[39]. While they are fantastic, I stopped half way (no disrespect) and hoped to finish them upon completion of the first reading of the *Gita*. I was hoping to learn the pre-meal prayer, however it remains work in progress.

Snacking between meals remains a challenge. I tried to get into an 'early-to-bed, early-to-rise' regime but lacked consistently. The carb-heavy diet during the final month was especially tough for me, perhaps by the end of it, I was too weary to experiment!

Some Learnings

Chaturmasa (coupled with *Gita* study), has been a fantastic experience, full of self-learnings, I summarize my top 3 themes here:

- *Sattva Aahar* – We eat more than we should eat (not sure where the three meals a day concept come from) and we eat things we should not be eating. Fruits and vegetables provide all the nutrition a human body requires, which can be supplemented by vegetarian food, with all its variety in terms of nutritious grains and spices and herbs and more – there are so many delightful dishes one can experiment with.

- *Chitta Shuddhi*[40] – Our scriptures are extremely powerful and are grounded in sound logic which most of us are ignorant about. They unravel so much about the cosmic universe. Reading, learning, understanding, chanting and assimilation of moral virtues – *daivi-sampad*[41] – in our daily life is a proven path to purify the mind.

- *Tapas* – *Sattva* lifestyle requires synchronization of the mind with the intellect and to calm our animal instincts through voluntary

---

39 https://youtu.be/3MRa2lR9MUg
40 Literally meaning, mental purity/mental cleanliness
41 Chapter 16 of *Gita, Daivasura sampad Vibhaga yoga* presents the categories of moral/ethical values that are useful to gain mental purity.

discipline and self-control. It involves alignment of 'thoughts, words and deeds' – *Arjavam*[42] – simply put, 'saying what you think and doing what you say'; of course, easier said than done!

Looking beyond Chaturmasa 2020

Chaturmasa is not a mere fasting ritual, it's a step towards gradually imbibing a way of life!

I hope to eat and live *Sattva*, enjoy food yet be dispassionate about it and generally avoid *Tamasic* foods like onions and chilies as well as processed foods as much as possible. I plan to do *falahar*[43] *Ekadasi* fasts (fruits only) through the year and learn new *slokas* from the *Gita* and other scriptures – like *Bhaja Govindam*[44]. Next *Chaturmasa*, I would consciously adjust my last month's diet to a more balanced one, learning from this years' experience.

I am still a novice but for those looking to do *Chaturmasa* in 2021, here are some pointers:

- do not think too much about the benefits of *Chaturmasa*, experience it for yourself. Do it together preferably with a few likeminded friends or family and you will not regret it.

- it is not a sprint, it's a marathon (think Test matches, not T20 to use a cricketing analogy), it requires perseverance and discipline – listen to your body, learn & adapt along the way based on your spiritual orientation and most importantly, enjoy it

- be honest to yourself, even if you have to swerve off the *sankalp*, do it mindfully and slowly come back to it, you are doing it for yourself and not to prove anything to anyone else

Spiritualism continues to have a more evolved meaning to me, feel blessed by the powers of creation!

---

42 The words, *Arjuna* and *Arjavam* come from the same root verb, and means 'straightforwardness'.

43 Falahar means, 'fruits as food', literally.

44 https://en.wikipedia.org/wiki/Bhaja_Govindam; written by Adi Sankaracharya. Also known as *moha-mudgara*.

Attachment to Detachment

Finally, *Chaturmasa* got over!

I don't know from where I got the idea that food is enjoyment. Before the start I knew very well that I have an intense attachment to food. Added to that I also indulged in alcohol. It was perhaps deep ingrained in me. Obviously, I started to eat more to enjoy more. But as one progresses in life, I realized food is not so important at all but still, the attachment lingers.

I was looking to break this mindset. Then *Chaturmasa* happened.

I moved from a state where 'food was important' at the dawn of the *Chaturmasa* to 'just food for survival' by the time I finished the five months. Attachment to food has gone away, and now I am left to consider food is just like air we breathe and water we drink. I no longer have an attachment to the type or taste of food. *Chaturmasa* was all about "Food just enough for thought". Although intellectually I understand the statement, still the mind tries to go into old grooves trying to get ice-cream or some sweet after food. I need to find solutions for my sweet tooth. Maybe I should do a cold turkey like I did with my coffee and tea habits.

Chaturmasa is more about the overall development of three things – body, mind and intellect. The moment the mind is free from attachment to food, the intellect becomes free to think on spiritual matters and meditation. Bodily health also improved noticeably.

I enjoyed fasting during *Ekadasi, especially Nirjala*. I am determined to continue *Ekadasi* by His grace. Every Thursday I am planning water fasting from Jan 1 2021. I also intend to fast once a week going forward and adjusting for *Ekadasi*. I also intend to include a lot more fresh vegetables than cooked ones.

Spiritually my focus was on meditation and listening to *Bhagavad Gita*. Meditation is to keep the spiritual current going throughout the day. But I realized that the moment I open my eyes, I tend to forget God. Hence, I tried meditating while keeping my eyes open. This helped in thoughts/

contemplation on God even during working hours. I revised *Bhagavad Gita* till chapter 3.

Healthwise, I found an all-round improvement. While I am not able to lose much weight, I dropped 5 kilos in five months. I still need to lose 5 more kgs. There were some days that I deviated and ate outside food. But I noticed that I was not as keen as before to enjoy outside food. I also had the attitude that it was also just 'food for survival' rather than enjoyment.

Finally, I think I can improve upon all the shortcomings in the next *Chaturmasa.*

Melting the Iceberg[45]

I am blessed to have completed my fourth year of *Chaturmasa* fasting. It has acquired a new meaning in my life. This year has been less about food but more about spiritual enhancement. I also seemed to have unknowingly assumed a new responsibility (which I am happy about) of coaching other friends who started their first *Chaturmasa* fasting this year. Initially, I was indeed a bit concerned if I was coaching them in the right way or not... but in the course of the first two weeks, the concern went away as I realized that the people who joined me are self-motivated and are very involved in their own spiritual development. So, my task became much easier – it was more of being a 'shortcut' to an answer they were looking for, than of a real coach who would handhold the newbies.

One of the tangible physical benefits I got out of *Chaturmasa* was that my right frozen shoulder that had very limited movement, due to repetitive stress injury (RSI) caused by overuse of computer devices went away! I reduced my weight by about 10lbs which was not new for me given the patterns of the past few years. Eating fresh, healthy and only as much as the body needs, helped me to sleep better, wake up fresh and importantly, made me a permanent 4AM person now! By consciously abstaining from receiving other inputs from social media, reducing entertainment time I was able to find quality time and it helped me to publish a book[46].

Within the first month, our discussions were centered more on spiritual topics and less on food – which was very encouraging for me because *Chaturmasa* is to be used as a God-given opportunity to 'turn on the heat' [*tapah*] on ourselves to melt the deep rooted wrong

---

45 Diary of Rajesh Sengamedu, http://linkedin.com/in/sengamedurajesh, https://happilyoga.com

46 Happiness beyond Mind| Rising above Helplessness, Conflicts and Choices https://www.amazon.com/dp/B08CNLMGYM/ref=dp-kindle-redirect?_encoding=UTF8&btkr=1

understanding of what life's goal is and to rid ourselves of the ignorance of what is real and unreal.

I want to explain the concept of self control [*tapah*] with an analogy of an iceberg. Let us assume we have a 'thinking iceberg' (or an iceberg that has a mind). Like our mind, only a little of it is visible (conscious) and most of it is hidden (subconscious, unconscious).

Let us say that just over ninety nine percent of the iceberg is underwater, invisible to us. In the ocean there are so many such icebergs and each one now thinks it is different from other icebergs and importantly all the icebergs may think they are different from the water they are all in. The reality is that icebergs are just water in a different form! However, the iceberg now experiences an illusion that does not correspond to reality of who it is. The illusion now gives rise to 'individuality' where none exists. There is no difference between water or iceberg of any shape, size.

One of the ways the illusion will go away is by 'melting the entire iceberg' so it now becomes one with the water around. In the same way, we have to 'melt' our mind by applying self-discipline and seeking out energy sources that can melt the mind to reveal our true Self.

The visible 1% of our mind can be melted through *karma yoga*, – spiritualizing our daily work with an attitude that we are not the 'doer' but just an instrument – a small cog in the big wheel of nature, doing our bit to keep the *chakra* of life.

The invisible 99% of our mind can be melted through *japa yoga* – chanting using a *mantra*. The repetition/chanting creates new grooves in the mind. Our subconscious has so many unknown characteristics, desires, intentions that propel us into action – even without our knowledge and *japa* (chanting) helps to re-align those towards the 'Real I' – the *Atma* or *Brahman*, which is what is our true nature – just like the water which is the true nature of the iceberg.

A *mantra* is no different than the deity it represents. Deity can be loosely translated as the principle of nature: each element of nature is represented by a mantra, for example, air is deified in a mantra called *'yam'*. Likewise, each principle of nature has a mantra: say of 'omnipresence' represented by *'Vishnu'* mantra, or the 'auspiciousness' represented by *'Shiva'* mantra. Irrespective of what mantra we use, it is sure to create new thought patterns in the mind.

1. I have new found love and appreciation for mangoes that nourished me in the first two months of *Chaturmasa* and dates and bananas that were critical for me to thrive in the last month.

2. I learnt that there are plenty of nutritious grains, lentils, fruits and other ingredients that can be used to cook sumptuous meals. I plan to eat *sattvic* foods as much as possible going forward.

3. *Chaturmasa* has changed how I view food; from being a live-to-enjoy-food (gourmand) kind of guy, I now eat-to-live. I plan to continue with two meals per day with a 'cheat' day – to eat outside and/or *non-sattvic* food – once every fortnight.

4. It is easier to drop bad habits (and inculcate good habits) when you are intensely focused on it. *Chaturmasa* provided me five months to do so and with *Daivam* and a supportive group like ours, it was fun too.

5. *Ekadasi* fasting is very spiritual if practiced regularly and with the right intent. Fasting with the group made it even better for me.

6. Our scriptures are full of deep insights, and *gyan* and *Vedantic* prescription – of *sravana, manana* and *nididhyasana*[47] – will help me deal with the ups and downs of this world effortlessly.

---

47 Literally, *listening, understanding* and *assimilating*. This is the process for self-transformation, using the scriptural knowledge about who we truly are, are not and what is our relationship with this world. In this process, we suspend our pre-conceived notions about what spirituality is/what the definition of our own self is and *listen attentively* to the teachings. Obviously, when the teachings do not align with our view of the world, we try to *understand* where the dissonance is and clarify that dissonance through further listening and or asking the *Guru* or peer groups (*satsang*). Finally, once we are convinced, the additional important step of *converting* that knowledge into assimilated knowledge makes for the complete transformation of who we are to who we truly are. This is also a good process for transactional worldly knowledge as well.

7. The mind is very difficult to control/dissolve and requires intense *tapah* over a long period of time; daily meditation is the key.

8. Having a *guruji* is essential for one's spiritual journey; however, one has to be very deliberate about finding him.

9. Chanting of the meal prayer verses is an important way to remind myself who I really am (not that I have realized it).

10. Lastly, the verse 30 from *Bhaja Govindam* [48]summarizes what I intend to practice for the rest of my life.

   a. *Breath control, sense control, reflection on the distinction between the eternal and ephemeral, practice of japa leading to samadhi (silence) — practise these with devotion, very carefully.*

May *Daivam* continue to guide us!

---

48 https://vedantavision.org/bhaja-govindam-verse-30/

If I Can, Anyone Can

In a few words – *Chaturmasa* is very, very hard! It is also one of the most physically and mentally beneficial endeavors I have taken up – even though I did not necessarily follow it to the 'T'.

By background, I belong to an uber foodie family, and in my 51 years, I have taken my quest to new heights of seeking out lavish, rich food from different parts of the world and overindulging it. The opportunity to pursue *Chaturmasa* dropped into my lap. In a year I started questioning my relationship and association with food and started studying the teachings of Gita in my uni-group led by one of the fellow practitioners. So when the idea of taking up *Chaturmasa* together in a group was suggested I did not have to think too hard. Nor did I build a do-or-die aspiration to this. I am not sure if I would have taken this up last year.

The first day was the *Ekadasi* fast – 36 hours without water and food was brutal. Before that day I had never gone longer than I slept without food and water. I did 24 hours without food, but drank water. No caffeine – which was difficult. But it worked. The first six weeks were great – I followed the instructions very much to the letter. And lost five kilos of weight in the process – felt an incredible burst of energy – all by eating less and simply! Then I slipped big time! Starting with a brief holiday to the English Coast – I went all out with fish & chips, ice-cream wine, and other no-nos. It took me the best part of two months to rebalance. I did however, continue with the bi-weekly *Ekadasi* fast every fortnight – graduating to 36 hours without food and water, and even building in a weekly 24 wet fast.

In the end, as with my yoga practice, my frame of reference of what is good for me in terms of food has shifted, and I feel nourished in terms of knowledge and body. I do feel that a new understanding of the world has opened up in front of me. In a word – I feel way more resilient than I ever have. Yet again, with pure serendipity, *Chaturmasa* has burned through my inhibitions and put a mirror to my desires and failings. There is much work to do, and I look forward to the next round next year. In the meanwhile, I am resolved to do a weekly fast, and follow *Ekadasi* every fortnight.

If there ever was a time for everyone to consider their habits and impact this has on our world, it is now. And If I can take up the quest – anyone and everyone can.

Vignettes from Monthly Musings

In this chapter, we present a summary of how the participants progressed every month. Every month, we documented our observations and these are presented as candidly as we could to help you learn about the experience of *Chaturmasa* for each of the five participants. Each para corresponds to a month of *Chaturmasa* diaries and we talk of how our relationship with food changed. There are other spiritual, emotional benefits experienced that we summarize in the final month summaries presented earlier. While we have edited the summaries for brevity, we have also shared in public domain the exact diaries as written by each of the participants as we progressed through the five months. You can find the link to the writeups here[49].

Discovering Spiritualism & Becoming a Seeker

I was hesitant to sign up for *Chaturmasa*, though the mind saw the rationale behind this time-tested observance, I was not entirely convinced; it felt like a good test of endurance and will-power but there was a slight worry about potentially experiencing low energy levels and feeling weak within, there were self-doubts if the *sankalp* could be sustained once the initial excitement wore off, but having weighed it all up, the intellect agreed to give it a go. Completing one month has been **immensely satisfying**, both in terms of training of the mind and how the body feels. The **body feels lighter and energetic** despite regular *yogasanas* and meditation as well as evening walks (and an occasional run, weather permitting). To begin with, food held centre-stage but that receded after a week or so. Eating half-stomach isn't easy, therefore the focus has been on not overeating which one tends to do if there is a long gap between meals! The *Ekadasi* fasts went somewhat surprisingly easier than expected, without much perceived physical discomfort. Overall, this past month has been about **moderating desires** (*santosham* or contentment) – the **physical body feels good and internal organs detoxed**. The experience is a step towards building *titiksha*[50] (forbearance) and *vairagya*[51] (dispassion), and the **motivation levels are actually higher than at the beginning!**

After starting off the second month with a feeling of foot-being-off-the-pedal, I had to remind myself of my *sankalp* of eating *sattvic* food besides continuing with 2 meals a day and focusing on portion control. Interestingly, I think my body has adapted to *Chaturmasa* regime to the extent that even a small indulgence brings about a heaviness. Post dinner cravings remain a challenge and I continue to work on it. On *Ekadasi* day in mid August, I went for a run which was a bad idea, it had me feeling drained and somewhat weak at bedtime and the following day. Out of curiosity, I observed the Jain holy week of *Paryushan* (*Ekadasi* to Ganesh Chaturthi), and focused on spiritual thoughts, and proactively sought blessings from my near and dear ones. I even connected on an impulse, with a friend after a few years who I had consciously wronged in the past and sought his forgiveness. I found the experience very powerful and liberating. *Yogasana*, meditation, and 10,000 steps/day have now become a

---

50 *Titiksha,* or forbearance is the attitude that everything is in a cycle of flux and we are bound to experience opposites in our life. For example, heat & cold, happiness & sadness, praise & criticism – all these come in pairs. When we experience one, the other is bound to come sooner or later. Therefore, there is no need to lament or be extremely happy when either occurs as the tide will change soon!

51 *Vairagya* is a tough concept to understand, therefore it is also a much misunderstood word in modern times. It does not mean letting go of one's responsibilities and marching into a forest or mountain tops, wearing a saffron robe to meditate! It is on the contrary an attitude which we develop being very objective about our relationship with the universe and how it corresponds to our happiness. When we know that the entire universe, including the objects, people, places, and even our own body & mind are constantly changing, therefore we do not need to be overly dependent on any of these to derive happiness. *Vairagya* is that state of recognition that we don't need to depend on any external 'things' including our mind for our happiness.

habit. Finally, yesterday I did my first ever truly *Nirjala Ekadasi*, which was an amazing feeling. I broke the 70kg goal. I hope to stay in the 69 – 70kg zone for the rest of *Chaturmasa*.

After 3 months, the body felt quite comfortable with the 'new normal', the transition from no-yogurt to no-milk was very seamless. Using a cricketing analogy, we are now in the 'middle overs', trying to consolidate after a decent start! While there is a nice rhythm, I have been unable to resist playing a 'few loose shots', but never too reckless and thankfully, I have survived them all. Listening to my body, I have made some adjustments to my diet and am less rigid during family occasions like birthdays! We ate out for the first time in over 6 months and had a great time. I noticed myself ordering mindfully, without being unnecessarily fastidious though! Listening to one of the spiritual talks, I came across an interesting context to fasting as a way to reassert our essential nature which is the divine spirit – *Atman* – as distinct from the body mind complex (and its desires). Hence fasting (for the body, like meditation for the mind) is a way to discipline and calm our animal instincts and experience our real Self. *Nirjala* (no water) *Ekadasis* has been a mixed bag. In the past, I haven't particularly enjoyed the after-experience, lack of sleep being the most prominent, though I put it down to the weather! Last *Ekadasi* went much better, I did my morning walk before the sun came up and had some warm water thereafter, which kept me going for the rest of the day.

The fourth month in this year's *Chaturmasa* also known as *Purushottam* month (*Adhika-masa*[52]) went relatively smoothly, the two meal routine is now a habit, though admittedly, there still are days when I have to deal with cravings. *Ekadasi* fasting has progressively gotten easier too, though I

---

52 Hindu calendars get adjusted once every four years – this concept of adjustment gives an 'extra' month once every four years, known as *adhika maasa*, literally meaning *extra month*. There is no presiding deity for this cosmological calculations, hence it is named after the Supreme Being, *Purushottama*. It is a tradition for Indian homes to donate money (& things like food stuff, clothes etc) during this month. Also, it is to be noted that in 2020, *Chaturmasa*, was for a duration of roughly five months, instead of the usual four because of this adjustment.

do drink some warm water – somehow I am not convinced about *Nirjala*! Last month, I also did Navratri fasting, eating fruits during the day and a *Sattvic* meal after sun-down. I now weigh a balanced 68kg, let's see for how long.

Religion and spiritualism now have a more evolved meaning to it, feel blessed by the powers of creation!

Physical to Mind Connection

I had chronic pain in my left calf muscle for at least 20 years and in the last 20 days I had no pain in the calf at all. That, I believe, is the result of fasting. I lost only 3 kgs in the first month. I feel meditation is possible only because the body is lighter now. I look forward to another four months of *Chaturmasa* and work on my meditation practice.

Eating twice a day became easy, but the challenge was 'after food'. As there was no yogurt this month, I found it difficult, coming from South India wherein yogurt is a must to end the platter. Naturally, the ending was a bit spicy and my mind was looking for something sweet. More than searching for something sweet it was my cravings in disguise. It was clear to me that these are simple cravings. Being conscious I was able to control sometimes and yielded to eating something sweet. Sweet, sometimes fruit and sometimes *kheer*, but continued the fasting routine without yogurt this month. I adopted a 'no eating policy' after 6 pm in the evening. Consequently, ended up most of the time having a good meal in the morning and fruits in the evening. I noticed that if the quantity of food in the morning is a little more, it makes me a bit dull especially if I have consumed rice. The mind was naturally calm, and this aided me in getting up early in the morning at 4.30 and meditating for one hour. I gradually progressed to observing *Nirjala Ekadasi*. My weight dropped a few kilos from 89/88 kg to 83/84 kg now. I hope to be 80 by September month-end.

I continued to eat twice daily with no milk this month. One big meal and small meal around 5.30/6.00 pm in the evening. From the third month it had become a routine. I became complacent and skipped meditation practice. Naturally, my mind craved processed food like chips. I also noticed that the more I meditated, I needed less sleep and less food. However, if my mind was disturbed, I ended up eating more food. Also, the more conscious I was about what I was eating, I ate less. **It was a big revelation: Food, sleep, processed food and meditation – all were interlinked**. I have noticed many benefits due to *Chaturmasa*. My physical health improved – GERD[53] – an issue I struggled with for years and chronic pain in my left leg went away. I started to wonder how much unwanted food like tea, biscuits, snacks I was munching on mindlessly earlier. I also observed that boredom made me eat! Finally, *sattvic* qualities like patience, perseverance started manifesting in me easily.

By the time the fourth month of *Chaturmasa* set in, I realized the power of mind over food. My notion that eating less food would impact my virility was proven false. Fasting on *Ekadasi* became very comfortable, and it felt as if the question paper was leaked before the exams – knowing what to do and following the script!

Living with Food to Subsist, Not Enjoy

I am fond of peanuts…and when I am bored I am tempted to eat peanuts. I resolved that this month I will eat just twice a day and nothing in between. Fortunately I was able to stick to my resolution. It shows that the mind is more powerful than our cravings. I read somewhere that when the 'cooking process' inside our stomach begins, it is best not to put more inside till the food is digested. I think it makes perfect sense. Healthy eating does NOT mean eating healthy food alone, it also means eating right! I am excited to share that the range of movement I did not have in my right shoulder (due to a frozen shoulder problem that has been going on for year) improved significantly in this month. I am now able to move my right arm a bit more freely. Other interesting data for you: I lost 5lb in one month

---

53 GERD – Gastroesophageal reflux disease which causes food to come up and leave a bad feeling, often choking the throat, and with breathing difficulties for a few seconds.

[155lb ->150lb], while continuing to average 7,000 steps a day (equal to roughly 3.2 miles/day). I noticed a consistent sleep pattern of ~6hours/day [10AM to 4AM].

Food has a direct bearing on how we feel. Eating food that increases *sattvic* energy content in the body is a spiritual practice that serious practitioners always follow. *Sattvic* does not mean vegetarian. It just means that there are specific foods (even amongst vegetarian fare) that we can eat and we cannot. For example, onions and garlic are known to arouse passion, energy, and an extroverted mind. Similarly, *moong dal* is known to evoke the *sattvic* constitution in the body. Since the last two months, I have avoided food that is *tamasic*, because it hinders gaining knowledge by making us lethargic – not just at a bodily level but also mentally. Our focus has been to increase the *sattva* content in the body so that the mind can be used appropriately to gain knowledge, read scriptures, meditate and to develop right values like *ahimsa* (non-violence), *satya* (speaking truth) etc. I stuck with eating just two square meals a day with no snacking in between meals. The food itself was a simple fare – usually quinoa with some *sambar* or other dish and a vegetable. I am now convinced that I was eating more than what my body needs. *Chaturmasa* is a great exercise to not only control the quantity of food but also our eating habits. I seem to have banished the word 'snack' from my dictionary. I feel more energetic, my body weighs a lot less, and my mind becomes extremely perceptive. I also noticed that except on one occasion when I was upset for a few minutes, I maintained a natural calm, peaceful disposition. Also, there were a few trying moments, when I could have slipped into a mode of 'violent thoughts' against somebody else, but I was able to consciously send 'gratitude' towards them. I am actually amazed at this change in my attitude. While I don't entirely attribute it to the *sattvic* food I am eating in this period, it is a combination of food, studies, meditation practice and in general a determined understanding that my goal is important and worth chasing, rendering those moments of anger, depression, violence powerless to influence me.

The third month has been uneventful. Or rather, it had become a routine to just look forward to eating two square meals a day – around 930AM and 4PM, nothing to eat or drink in between, except water. The *Nirjala-Ekadasi* that I did last month was interesting – it seems to have become the new normal: fasting once every fortnight seems to have become easier. I lost 9lb in 3 months. Here are FIVE THINGS I did for the last three months. I have ordered them in the increasing order of difficulty levels to practice. I recommend you to try even one or two below and discover the benefits. Other than the physical benefit of weight loss, you may also experience several mental & emotional benefits.

a. Stopped eating leftovers, frozen food, microwaved food

b. Stopped eating any sort of processed food. If I did not understand any of the ingredients or found 'chemical-sounding' names (including the innocuous ascorbic acid) in the packaging, I considered that as packaged food

c. Stopped snacking in between meals. Ate just twice in 24 hours with a gap of ~5–6 hours, and just water in between.

d. Ate only when I was hungry and reduced food quantity to approximately half to three-fourths of what I normally eat.

e. Fasting once a fortnight: No solids for ~36 to 40 hours (5 pm the day before the fast, to 9 am the day after fast); and no water too for ~24 hours (6 pm of the previous day to 6 pm on the day of fast), out of that 36 hours: called *nirjala Ekadasi* in *Sanskritam*. [one can adapt according to their body – maybe drink water/milk/eat fruits etc., on the day of fast...]. I am a lacto-vegetarian but I see no reason why the above should not work even for non-vegetarians.

In the fourth month, I stayed on course to eat when hungry. Personally, I set out to rid myself of the habit of eating when bored and eat only hungry. By the Divine's grace I was successful just eating two square, simple, small meals a day, usually between 9–10AM and later at 230–430PM. Interestingly, this month, on several days, I ended up eating the same stuff both times – which was a big improvement for me as I was consciously reducing the 'options' I had to eat. My attitude had changed towards the second meal – was not looking for variety and was happy to eat the same stuff as morning. Like we see in nature, variety is beautiful but creating a variety of food items to consume takes time, energy (and money). Importantly, seeking out variety is an indication of an extraverted mind that is looking for entertainment, or is bored or just imaginative! Nothing wrong with consuming different types of food and I encourage all to do it, but the purpose of *Chaturmasa* for me was different – it was to 'get over' the dependence on (tasty) food and transcend the 'need' for (tasty) food. The objective was to be happy with whatever one gets to eat!

In the fifth month, because of the 'no *dal*' (lentils) rule – no dicotyledons or polycotyledons in this month, I struggled with balanced food, till I discovered red matta rice which has roughly the same amount of proteins as in dals – 9 grams proteins per 100 grams, and substituted for lack of lentils in the food consumed during the month. This month saw an increase in consumption of bananas & dates (which were the only fruits allowed, an occasional mango too), milk, yoghurt and paneer. Thanks to the group & also my wife's innovative ideas, I enjoyed a variety of *dosas* with different types of flours mixed into them – ragi, rice, wheat, barley etc., I continued with my strict two meal diet a day, skipping dinners on all days. Usually, I ate around 9–10AM in the morning followed by another meal between 3–5PM in the evening and just water in between. I am hoping to make it a habit to eat just twice a day with no mindless snacking! *Nirjala Ekadasi* [i.e fasting without food, water] has been difficult for me. I tried earnestly every *Ekadasi* but my body is not yet ready to adapt.

Power of *Sankalp and* Hedonism to Spiritualism

Hindu scriptures talk about taking care of one's health for one's spiritual growth. It is said that one who can't voluntarily give time for his or her health will have to forcibly give time to diseases. This notion appealed to me. Therefore, my personal objective in the first month of *Chaturmasa* was to adopt certain dietary restrictions and eat *sattvic* food, so that my mind and body were more receptive to spiritual knowledge. It has been a transformative month in which lots of my assumptions and beliefs were tested & discarded. One of my favorite maxims comes from a play by Oscar Wilde: "I can resist everything but temptations". Prior to following the prescribed dietary restrictions, I thought it would be almost impossible to survive without eating ANY vegetables for the entire month, and at some point, I thought I would succumb to the temptation. However, I was not tempted as much as I expected. Giving up certain foods and being able to lead a better-than-normal life has made me discard this belief in my own limitations. Having eaten only two meals per day – breakfast & lunch – for the past few weeks and being equally productive, if not more so than the previous months, I can tell you that it is not as difficult as I used to believe. All I needed was a *Chaturmasa sankalp* and a support system of my spouse, other family members, and fellow *Chaturmasis*.

My strange addiction to tea reduced drastically from a daily intake of six cups, I am down to only one cup per day thanks to an anti-tea concoction. Previously, I would have been shaken by the very thought of not drinking even a sip of water throughout the day. All my *Ekadasi* fasts had plenty of fluids throughout the day – water, herbal tea & coconut water. On a whim, I decided to go for it yesterday and folks, with his divine grace, I did not eat or drink anything for 30+ hours! During my yoga sessions, I can now do certain asanas easily that I had always found hard to do previously. In certain breathing exercises, I can hold my breath for longer, effortlessly. My mind was so receptive that I was able to memorize a few *slokas* very quickly & they will become part of my morning rituals for life.

The second month was much easier than the first month for a number of reasons: my body had completely adjusted to thriving on fewer meals, each with smaller portion sizes; vegetables returned to my plate and hence offered me a bit more variety; and lastly, I had learnt to enjoy *sattvic* foods. In the middle of the month, I ate fast-food – to celebrate my son's birthday – for the first time after almost five months. Although I enjoyed eating this food, I didn't feel that I had missed it. I was pleasantly surprised to find that a few months of eating home-cooked meals and the last eight weeks had led to a 'taste-*vairagya*'. **Where before I used to live to eat, now I just eat for nourishment – the transformation is complete!** In the third week of this month, I decided to do a 5-day detox, which meant that I only ate raw vegetables and fruits for two days and juices for the other three days. Surprisingly, I was very energetic and productive during those days. However, my weight dropped quite a bit by the end of the detox, which bothered my family members. To correct, I increased the portion sizes of my meals in the last week. One of the best things that happened to me this month was that I completely got over my habit of drinking four to six cups of tea daily. By the end of the first month, I was down to one cup, but since the first week of August, I have been completely off tea and don't miss it. Equally important, I don't need any concoction to control my tea-urges. Having memorized two meal prayer verses and assimilated their beautiful meanings, I can tell you that food has acquired a new meaning for me. Beyond taste and satisfying hunger pangs, it has become an expression of gratitude and an offering to God and in turn to oneself. What's the meaning of this prayer, you may ask. As I understand it, at one level, the verses are chanted to cleanse food from impurities, but on a deeper level, as Swami Sarvapriyanandaji explained in one of his discourses, the verses are all about acknowledging Brahman in the entire process. Inspired by my first *Nirjala* (without water) *Ekadasi* fast last month, I decided to continue with the practice this month as well. It is not easy to go without water or food for 30–36 hours continuously, but somehow, divine grace is always there to support one's such *sankalps*, and that's when one learns to acknowledge the presence of a higher being – a being that is inside oneself and guides everything.

The third month was volatile with higher "highs" and lower "lows". Among the "lows": for the first time I ate a packet of *namkeen*, a snack readily available in most Indian households, that is exactly the type of processed food one is supposed to avoid during this period. I had opened the *namkeen* packet before I started *Chaturmasa*, and, upon seeing the impending expiry date, my strong belief in not wasting food won over my conviction to practice 'dhamah' (sense control). I ate it on two consecutive afternoons to finish the packet off. Fortunately, I did not enjoy it. To avoid such internal conflict again, I promptly gave away the unopened *namkeen* packets in our house. As they say in Hindi: *na rahega baas, na bajegi basuri* (roughly translated – if there is no flute, then there will not be any music). The second of the "lows" was that I ate *non-sattvik* food twice during the last 28 days. I went out to meet a friend (who was visiting from the US), and I ate at a restaurant, (appropriately named *Annamaya*, I might add!), for the first time in the last six months. Although the food was tasty, I did not enjoy the experience. The end result was predictably not good. Fortunately, I was able to overcome a bloated stomach and other such side effects through a brisk walk, digestive drink and yoga class the next day. The second incident was at my birthday, where I permitted myself, ahead of time, to enjoy a celebratory meal with the family. Another "low" was that my food portions at lunch meals have steadily increased during the last month. While I still eat only two meals during the day, the amount of food has certainly increased. I realized during this month that I tend to lose weight readily if I try to cut back on my food intake. My goal of bringing down my weight to 68 kgs morphed into keeping my weight in the 65–67 kgs band and therefore, I decided to avoid strict portion control. I also experienced some of the higher "highs" I experienced during the last month. My body showed increased flexibility, and I was able to do certain yogic asanas (e.g. *chakra asana*) which I hadn't even attempted since my school days. I plan to get better at some of the other asanas that have eluded me (e.g. *Halasana*). I was a bit adventurous with my *Ekadasi* fasting and decided to increase the number of hours I fasted (without food or water) on both occasions. Diving into reading spiritual books and chanting made it easier for me to abstain from water and food.

Inspired by my *co-chaturmasis* ruminations on the health benefits of their *Chaturmasa* experiences, I also reflected on how the last few months has improved my health. I have been able to kick my habit of drinking 4–6 cups of tea daily and I have replaced it with healthier drinks. Another clear, observable benefit is that I have lost over 10 kgs and therefore, I am able to do several yogic asanas that I used to find very difficult to perform.

My body has increasingly become more flexible than ever. While I haven't visited an optometrist (and don't plan to until the end of the pandemic), I did observe an improvement in my eyesight. I am now able to work without my spectacles during most days. I also reached a personal goal for my *Ekadasi* fasting – with divine blessings, I fasted for 48 hours without water or food. It was rough going at times but by having faith, listening to spiritual discourses, becoming more introspective, practicing *pranayama*, and resting as necessary, I was able to see myself through the two day fast. A few months ago, I would be petrified at the thought of *nirjala* (without water) *Ekadasi* fasting, but with the strict discipline of the *Chaturmasa* diet, the idea of testing my limit (of going without food or water) somehow became very alluring. Since then, I continued to increase the hours of abstinence on each *Ekadasi* fast, building up stamina for the last fast. On the downside, I was less productive at work on *Ekadasi*; therefore, I have decided to limit my fasting to 36 hours going forward. I struggled with my urges for *non-sattvic* food in the last week. I found myself dreaming about some snacks (like *samosas*) that have been off my meal plate since March! The last four months have been transformative in my understanding of the body-mind complex with support of my fellow *chaturmasis* and *Gita* Group members. Spiritualism is gradually becoming a way of life for me with eating only *two-sattvic* meals a day, meditating (as subpar as it is), focusing on introspection, listening to *Bhaj Govindam* and discourses, and learning from our scriptures. The next challenge is to incorporate more of *Bhagavad Gita*'s core teachings into my daily life.

Ups & Downs but Sticking to the Plan

For the first time in my 50+ years of life I have managed to stick to the regime – and fasted for longer than the time I slept – twice, in fact! Yet again, it never ceases to amaze me how the mind creates these dependencies and inhibitions, and how easily it is possible to burn through this! I dealt with nasty headaches – withdrawal symptoms from coffee, which I love, and was really not sure I would make it through day 1, the first *Ekadasi* fast. I fasted 24 hours instead of 36 and it was frankly, a struggle. And I did not realize I missed green vegetables so much! I also fell off the wagon on the fourth day – eating three double scoops of chocolate ice-cream! I have since built-in having a fruit salad or sorbet during the day between lunch and dinner. Though I did manage to go to raucous BBQ and not have any meat or alcohol. The second fast of 36 hours was easier – because I knew it would end, and there was food within arms-reach. The caffeine withdrawal took eight days – as before. Having stuck with it for the last four weeks, I am starting to see the possibility of a lifestyle change, where food does not rule my mind and life. I have naturally drifted into a routine of sleeping early – latest 10 pm, and rising early (4.30 – 5.00 am) – followed by a couple of hours of mind/body nourishment including prayer, meditation, pranayama breathing, walk or Ashtanga yoga, yin stretches and reading before starting the day. I have been fairly good at keeping meals to 9 am – 7 pm, and I have managed an evening walk 4 times a week as well. Most important is that none of this feels like a chore or something that is finite. Lots more energy, and I even dropped 4+ kg of weight. Long may this continue.

I completed my fifth *Ekadasi* fast and first *nirjala* fast a day earlier on Friday. My earlier mid-August fast involved two glasses of water mid-day. No cravings, no need to sleep during the day, and I continued with two 5K/day walks as well – the second one just before breaking the fast yesterday. Unlike previous fasts, I was actually looking forward to this. Some sort of salvation. Barring the two fasts, August has been a forgettable month. I questioned the fast and its benefits for much of the first half, and slipped several times, indulging in sweets and ice-cream, and even taking a glass of wine. This was nothing compared to last weekend while vacationing on the coast with my family! I could not resist the temptation of fine food and wine. I had coffee and ice-cream, fish and wine every day for five days. I have not felt the temptation for this entire year, but somehow this time it got the better of my best judgement. Truthfully I did not feel guilty doing this, but I have been mentally kicking myself most of the last week. Coffee withdrawal compounded the sluggishness and lethargy. Feeling great today, and I find myself at a crossroads, and not sure I am worthy to continue the diet.

This is the second month of drifting for me. It goes to show it is not as easy as many of my fellow practitioners make it look. I have not managed two meals a day, nor have I managed to stay away from milk (dairy version). Which is bemusing, in that I do not suit dairy. My milk intake is through ice-cream, which I do not seem to let go. Quantities and exercise are ok overall, as my weight has dropped modestly over the last month. I do enjoy the *Ekadasi* fast – even look forward to it. No problem with '*nirjal*' – no water for 36 hours and still manage to do 5k walks, thrice. So much so that I have resolved, and implemented, a weekly fast in-between the *Ekadasi* fasts – a wet 24 hour fast. Love it for the energy, calm and feeling of completeness it brings. As to the rest of the fast, rather than guilt, my dominant sense is of bemusement and feeling incomplete. I know and understand the context and relevance of *Chaturmasa*; but there is a blockage somewhere in the acceptance of this. This is something to work on. The goal for this month is to not eat after 5 pm, and step away from ice-cream.

Basically, after three months of yogurt and milk abstinence (which are really not in my regular diet), and having taken a detour via a real binge of ice cream during September and early October (although I have been on the wagon for the last three weeks!) I find myself some distance behind the plan and intent of *Chaturmasa*. The ice-cream cravings were really googly, as milk is not really in my diet. However, the revelations of how I associate with food, and the role food plays, or should play, have been revealing.

Much work to do, but a plan is emerging.

The *Chaturmasa* Workbook

Here is a ready reckoner[54] of the *Chaturmasa* guidelines we followed during 2020. **Notice that in this year, the duration was five months instead of four months.** The live version of the ready reckoner will be changed every year with updated instructions, dates and tips & suggestions as more people experience the power of *Chaturmasa* to transform themselves into happy & healthy individuals. If you follow the above ready reckoner link you can download the 2021 *Chaturmasa* updated guidelines and dates.

The Basic Plan: Physical Body Management – Foods to Eat, Foods to Avoid

AVOID/ ALLOWED	*1 Jul – 29 Jul (M1)*	*30 Jul – 28 Aug (M2)*	*29 Aug – 26 Oct (M3)*	*27 Oct – 26 Nov (M4)*
AVOID	All green leafy vegetables (If you can, avoid ALL vegetables)	Yoghurt/Curds [But you must consume 'thin' buttermilk to reduce dry skin symptoms]	Milk/Milk Products	All types of *dal* (lentils), especially those that can be split into two or having many seeds – like groundnuts, peas, beans (dicotyledons, polycotyledons)

---

54 We will update the ready reckoner here every year. Please bookmark this page. You are free to download this and adapt to your needs: https://docs.google.com/spreadsheets/d/1D5L-jQXA9pMl1JZeshekbLj4B0hw_jFJvmBfJggBIcw/edit#gid=0

AVOID	All processed food like cheese, bakery products; All sorts of stimulants – tea, coffee, alcohol; All non-vegetarian foods incl. eggs, chicken, seafood, meat No leftovers [ideal is to cook & eat freshly prepared food daily] Onions, Garlic, Green Chilies
ALLOWED	Anything else that is vegetarian other than what is listed for the month. When you run out of ideas, make Khichdi. In the months when you can eat Yoghurt/Curds, always dilute it to make butter-milk and drink/eat

Legend: M1= Month 1 & so on.

While more research needs to be done on the scientific basis of this practice, we are presenting the plan we followed in 2020 that resulted in wonderful benefits for every one of us.

Enhanced Basic Plan:
Physical Body Management – Portion Control

# Meals per day	Not more than 3 times in a day. If you can, eat dinners before 6pm OR at least 3 hours before you go to bed **Eat ONLY when you are hungry.** **If you are not hungry, skip a meal BUT don't eat out of habit.** **Avoid snacking in between if you can.** If you cannot avoid snacking, choose fresh fruits, & dry fruits, milk (adhere to quantity restrictions at all times and avoid milk in third month (M3), and shifting to butter-milk instead

Yogic tradition says,

- if we eat two times a day, we are *yogi* (i.e., who meet our physical body needs),

- if we eat three times a day, we are *bhogi* (i.e., someone who is an enjoyer)

- if we eat four times a day, we are a *rogi* (i.e., someone who is likely to fall sick soon)

- if we eat five times a day, we are a *drohi* (someone who is a greedy person, and eating someone else's food)

Quantity per meal	Half your stomach full; Usually, this is equal to two handfuls of food. But vary the quantity based on your body needs. Arrive at the right quantity after a few days of experimentation. Sip water as needed while eating. Quarter stomach full for water and leave a quarter empty

We don't recognize it but we end up over-eating. Science talks of 2000–2200 calories/day for an adult. Calories calculation apart, the science of Ayurveda suggests this proportion – half stomach full solids, quarter stomach full liquids and quarter empty for digestive processes to release air;

The rough quantity of solids that you need to take is 2 'anjana' measures. The measure one 'anjana' is equal to the amount of solids that both your hands can hold. [Be reasonable! Don't pile it up:-)].

Sleep & Exercise	Set up a regular sleep schedule and stick to it. You must be able to exercise regularly – at least 30–40min without feeling any strain.

Sleep is absolutely necessary for recuperative body functions. Setting a regular schedule trains the body to expect the required rest it needs daily.

Any sort of exercise is required to be done daily – be it yoga, gym, walking, jogging/running.

Advanced Plan: Subtle Body Management

for Pranic (Energy) Body (*Pranamaya Kosha*)	To- Do's [To balance physiological functions of the body]	If you would like, do 3 alternate nostril breathing (without breath retention) before every meal. Or at least 10 min of alternate nostril breathing every day, preferably in the morning. But surely say a small prayer to thank the bountiful nature for the food on the plate. Say a prayer[55] – offering everything that you eat to that Supreme Principle. We recommend you learning meaning and memorizing these two slokas from *Bhagavad Gita*: http://www.sathyasai.org/about-us/health-corner/food-prayer

The five physiological functions of respiration, digestion, elimination (of waste), circulation (of nutrients through the bloodstream) and reversal (special processes like coughing, sneezing, etc.) are balanced through alternate nostril breathing. Yogic tradition says that there are five subdivisions of prana, (life force) known as *prana, apana, samana, vyana, and udana* who control the entire body processes.[56]

Alternate nostril breathing before eating your meal stabilizes these five energies inside the body and helps in these physiological processes.

---

55 You would have noticed in the practitioners diaries, about the significance of the prayers before a meal. It is very similar to saying 'grace' before a meal. The deeper philosophical meanings behind the two specific meal prayers we followed (as in the link above) have convinced us that the subtler energy in the food we eat is the very source of our mind's energy and it can be enhanced with a prayer, acknowledging not just the 'farm to fork' chain, but even those forces of nature, without which the food will be an impossibility!

56 For an excellent understanding of the power of breath, please refer to Swami Niranjananda's book, Prana and Pranayama, published by Bihar School of Yoga, Munger, India: https://www.amazon.com/Prana-Pranayama-Swami-Niranjanananda-Saraswati/dp/8186336796

for Emotional Body (*Manomaya Kosha*)	To- Do's [Attitudes towards food & other sensory inputs]	Eat silently, slowly, with your entire attention on the food you are eating. Do at least 20min of daily meditation – stick to the same time, same place, same practice every day as far as possible. Have an attitude of respect towards the food, and remember that this is what is nourishing you. Reduce other sensory inputs – especially watching TV (like senseless soaps) or social media. Restricting wasteful use of water: by reducing the duration of shower for example.

You will need to follow this step IF your expected benefit is beyond the physical health. These practices introduce the centering of your mind, and help you to develop an attitude of respect towards the food. This attitude will change our approach towards food. It is similar to the attitude we will have towards a relationship: nurture a relationship because we care; and make it transactional because we don't care. Our attitude of 'caring' is all it takes to nurture something or not!

for Intellectual Body (*Vignanamaya Kosha*)	To-Do's [To sharpen the intellect]	Spend 30 min a day to read: any autobiography of a person that inspires you OR Any sort of spiritual literature – anything that would inspire you; anything that you always wanted to do but put off. If you cannot find anything, listen to spiritual discourses, especially **Bhagavad Gita.** YouTube has many such discourses that are free.

Body has just one way to gain its nutrients – through the mouth.

But the mind has five ways – hearing, smelling, seeing, touching, tasting. This practice is to help the mind not diverge and to calm down & settle down.

Common Obstacles & Recommendations

Some Obstacles & How to Overcome	If you get headaches & you crave for tea/coffee – sip hot water or hot milk If you feel hungry & the quantity of food is less – increase the quantity If you travel – ignore the restrictions in this sheet but try to adhere as closely as you can. You feel agitated because you have more time on hands now – Read a book, listen to an enriching podcast or meditate. If you are not sure how to identify processed food – go with a simple rule: if any ingredient sounds like a chemical, then avoid those. If on some days you feel like 'cheating' on the rules – it is perfectly fine. Be conscious of your decisions though. If you crave sweets – eat jaggery or dates or fruits. One of the favorite sweet-dishes we enjoyed was mashing all of those up together with a dash of ghee and dry fruits sprinkled on it.
Few Recommendations	Drink plenty of warm water. Avoid cold water/ice. You can add turmeric & black pepper to hot milk and make it a nice drink. Half a teaspoon of turmeric for 200ml of milk and a pinch of pepper. Use pepper, ginger, turmeric, cumin, fennel seeds/powder in your cooking to add flavor to cooked food. Don't use any sort of *masala*/spices that are pre-mixed [like *sambhar masala powder* from the stores] Switch to brown sugar or jaggery, Himalayan rock salt

Recipes

We recommend that you create your own recipes using simple ingredients. However, to inspire you with a few ideas, we share a few popular guidelines here from our *Chaturmasa* 2020 experience here.

We strongly recommend trying red *matta* rice or quinoa instead of standard, white long grain rice or basmati rice. Of course, you can always change what you eat based on how bored you are of a particular grain. These have enough proteins and nutrients for our bodies.

For those who have a sweet tooth, try mashing dates (or raisins, dry figs), bananas, honey, jaggery together with a dash of ghee and eat after your meal. This will be a satisfying sweet dish that is simple to make and healthy to consume. You can add roasted cashews for enhancing taste.

Ensure that you are eating enough freshly available fruits – especially mangoes. They are not only nutritious; they are filling as well.

Elsewhere in this book, we have shared references to a couple of websites that we have looked up for food recipes. Government of India, Ministry of Health portal which we reference here has several recipes. However, please choose only those that fit the restrictions as per the month during *Chaturmasa.*

The bottom line is, one should be brave and remove any concerns (which will play like devils inside our doubting minds) if we are getting adequate nutrients or not. The *Chaturmasa* system does NOT measure calories consumed or nutrients in the form of proteins, carbohydrates, minerals, lipids or vitamins. On the contrary, the regimen expects you to consume more of *sattvic* foods, some *rajasic* foods and avoid *tamasic* foods.

To help you with the categorization (*guna*) of various foods in *sattvic, rajasic & tamasic* categories, we provide a ready reckoner in this chapter.

Month 1 – Abstaining from All Vegetables

Liberally use spices, cumin seeds, black whole pepper and lentils (*chana dal*) -slightly dry roasted on slow flame and powdered finely. Mix with rice, *ghee* (clarified butter), and salt to taste.

Eat rice, *chapati* (Indian bread) with various types of lentils. Lentils can be used in two different forms – boiled, roasted & powdered.

Try different varieties of *dosas* (Indian style crepes) and use powdered lentils with ghee as a side dish. You can also alternate using yoghurt instead of ghee along with powdered lentils.

Yoghurt, *paneer* (cottage cheese) based dishes are excellent sources of proteins. For example you can try *kadi* (the North Indian way) or *palidya* (South Indian *kadi,* without any vegetables). Or you can try *paneer* based dishes. Just use your imagination to make these *paneer* dishes.

Ghee is an excellent source of nutrients. In fact, the Western food magazines claim this to be a superfood!

Experiment with horse gram, black gram, kidney beans (*rajma*), chickpeas (*chhole*). Simplest way to cook is to boil lentils in a pressure cooker and garnish with oil and mustard/cumin seeds as per your preference.

If you are running out of ideas, *khichdi* is the all-time favorite. It is a mixture of equal measure of rice and lentils (yellow *dal*) and pressure cooked along. Once cooked, garnish using spices and for variety, use cashews as well in the garnishing.

Months 2, 3 – Abstaining from Yoghurt (Month 2), Milk (Month 3)

Firstly remember that in the month yoghurt is to be avoided, you can use milk and other forms of milk derivatives (*paneer* etc.). Likewise, in the month when milk is to be avoided, you can use yoghurt – but this has to be watered down significantly (say 1:5 proportion with water).

As vegetables get back on the menu this month, you will not face many challenges for ideas on what to cook!

Month 4 – Abstaining from Lentils

If you use red rice and root vegetables (which are allowed in this month) you will have ample varieties of recipes. Bring in coconut in various forms – dry, fresh, or powdered.

Try making *dosas* without any lentils. This is known as *'neer dosa'* (literally meaning water-*dosa*) which is very popular in the Karnataka region of India.

Food Category ('*Guna*')

The following table shows the three categories of food. This table has been reproduced verbatim from the book, Practical Lessons in Yoga by Swami Sivananda [57] (https://www.dlshq.org/download/practical.htm)

Sattvic foods

- Cow's milk, cream, cheese, butter, curd, ghee,

- All sweet fruits like: apples, bananas, grapes, papaya, pomegranates, mangoes, oranges, pears, peaches, pineapples, guavas, figs,

- Vegetables like coconut, brinjals, potatoes, cabbages, spinach, tomatoes, cucumber, pumpkin, cauliflower, okra, dried peas, lemon

- Dry fruits like almonds, pistachios, raisins, dates,

- Wheat, red rice, unpolished rice, barley, oat-meal, green-gram, bengal gram, green pulse, groundnuts,

- Sugar-candy, dried ginger, honey

Rajasic foods

- Fish, eggs, meat,

- Salt, chilies, asafetida,

- Pickles

- Tamarind, carrots, turnips

- Mustard & spices

---

57 https://www.dlshq.org/download/practical.htm; https://www.amazon.com/Practical-Lessons-Yoga-Swami-Sivananda/dp/817052010X

- Sour things, Hot things

- Tea, coffee, cocoa, white sugar

Tamasic foods

- Onion, garlic

- Beef, pork

- Tobacco

- Rotten things, stale things, unclean things, foods that are cooked twice

- All intoxicants like wine, liquors, drugs

Epilogue – An Idea to Eradicate World Hunger

Approximately 700 million go hungry daily in the world today. If a billion people sign up to the idea based on fasting & eating healthy we can easily afford to get these 700M people two square meals a day and improving holistic health simultaneously. The participants who sign up, will lead a healthy lifestyle leading to an overall increase in happiness quotient at individual (micro) level as well as at society (macro) levels.

Here is an idea worth considering:

Food scarcity can be eliminated if we combine three levers through an app:

1. Educating consumers about healthy living habits and encourage them to adopt these habits. The education can be provided in the form of short videos other educational content on the app.

2. Enabling consumers track their newly discovered healthy living habits (through lever 1). The habit tracking and dashboard is a way for the consumer to see how his plan is being put into action.

3. Donating money saved due to their new habits adopted to those suffering food scarcity. The money can be donated to any syndicated organizations like Diya Ghar, Second Harvest Food Bank or local religious institutions where they donate food to the needy.

Here is how the app will work:

1. Provide educational content about fasting, benefits of eating healthy – especially cutting down # of times people eat/day, moving from meat to vegetarian, fortnightly fasting

2. Encourage people to sign up and try new food habits for a month or so.

3. Baseline what they eat, how much, how often, approximate monthly food spend.

4. Daily enable them to track their daily eating habits – how often, how much food, approx. $ spent and show how much they are saving. Provide a comparable calorie count as well

5. At the end of their chosen period, they can choose to donate a portion or all of the money thus saved by living a healthier lifestyle to a food charity of their choice. The app will provide them a list of food charities for donation.

We share a broad level calculations of how we can solve world hunger problem:

If a person fasts on *Ekadasi* and eats 2 meals a day on other days, the $ saved will be:

- Assume, cost of a meal: $5

- Money saved from 3 to 2 meal/day: $5/day = $150/month

- Money saved on 2 *Ekadasi* in a month: $30/month

- Total money saved per person/month: $180

- Assuming operational food procurement & operational efficiency (at scale) will bring in an additional savings equivalent to 30%, the total money saved through fasting while living healthily is $180*1.3 = $234.

According to USDA[58], $234 will provide food for a family of five for a little under a week! Or, it is approximately feeding one person for a month with the savings from the food not consumed!

Finally, fasting and eating healthy, fresh foods is a simple idea that brings us into harmony with nature. Over time, when we adopt fasting in our lives, we are being truly inter-dependent on nature by being conscious of the environment. This itself will restore the much-needed ecological balance that can have positive long term effects on society and mankind.

Be the change you want to see in this world

– Mahatma Gandhi

We encourage any of you to reach out to us if you are inspired by this idea of solving world hunger. We would need people of different skills, from different walks of life to make that vision a reality. We invite you to work with us and flesh this idea out into a simple to use, intuitive application that millions may use to make lasting life-style changes and at the same time, alleviating world hunger. Our idea has merit but it is also audacious and needs not just technical skills to develop the application, but an entire ecosystem of partners who believe they can play a part – big or small to bridge the gap between hungry people and food.

---

58 https://www.usatoday.com/story/news/nation/2013/05/01/grocery-costs-for-family/2104165/

References

We encourage the reader to browse through the following website links that have been useful for us to formulate a *Chaturmasa* plan:

1. Check the blog for monthly musings of *Chaturmasa* participants

   a. http://happilyoga.com

2. For good recipes

   a. https://sites.google.com/site/harshalarajesh/recipees-for-chaturmasa
   b. https://ayushportal.nic.in/pdf/Food_Recipes_From_AYUSH.pdf

3. Articles on *Chaturmasa*

   a. https://en.wikipedia.org/wiki/Chaturmas
   b. https://www.sanatan.org/en/a/303.html

4. *Chaturmasa* from *Puranas* & scientific perspective

   a. http://madhwamrutha.org/chaturmasya-vrata/

5. Practical Lessons in Yoga by Swami Sivananda,

   a. https://www.dlshq.org/download/practical.pdf

6. To understand the concept of time that is different for living beings on earth and celestial beings and some insights into the 'pre-big bang' time

   a. https://happilyoga.com/2020/06/21/concept-of-time-creation-in-eastern-science/